Penelope,
Best Wishes on
your 21st Birthday
♡ Katrina Dearling
🅧🅧

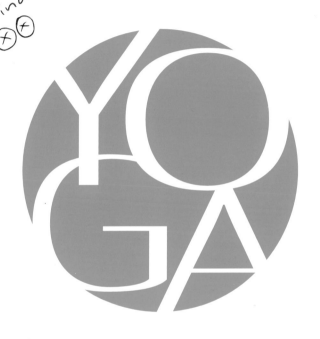

Some of the postures contained in this publication should only be attempted under the supervision of an experienced yoga practitioner. If in doubt, please contact your doctor or local yoga centre.

HarperCollins*Publishers*

First published in Australia in 1999
by HarperCollins*Publishers* Pty Limited
ACN 009 913 517
A member of the HarperCollins*Publishers* (Australia) Pty Limited Group
http://www.harpercollins.com.au

HarperCollins*Publishers*
25 Ryde Road, Pymble, Sydney, NSW 2073, Australia
31 View Road, Glenfield, Auckland 10, New Zealand
77-85 Fulham Palace Road, London W6 8JB, United Kingdom
Hazelton Lanes, 55 Avenue Road, Suite 2900, Toronto, Ontario M5R 3L2
and 1995 Markham Road, Scarborough, Ontario M1B 5M8, Canada
10 East 53rd Street, New York NY 10022, USA

National Library of Australia Cataloguing-in-Publication data:

Chapman, Jessie.
Yoga: postures for your body, mind and soul.
Includes index.
ISBN 0 7322 6547 9.
1. Yoga. I. Title.
613.7046

Cover: Rachel Hull in *Eka Pada Rajakapotasana*
Cover photograph by Jessie Chapman
All internal photographs by Dhyan
Printed in Australia by Griffin Press Pty Ltd on 115gsm New Era Satin

5 4 3 2 1   99 00 01 02 03

JESSIE CHAPMAN

YOGA

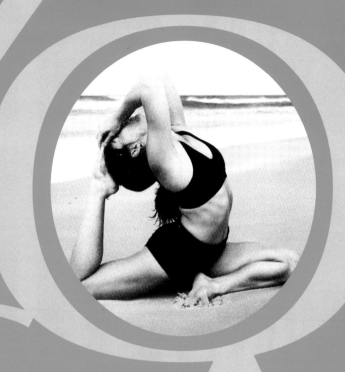

Postures for your body, mind & soul

HarperCollins*Publishers*

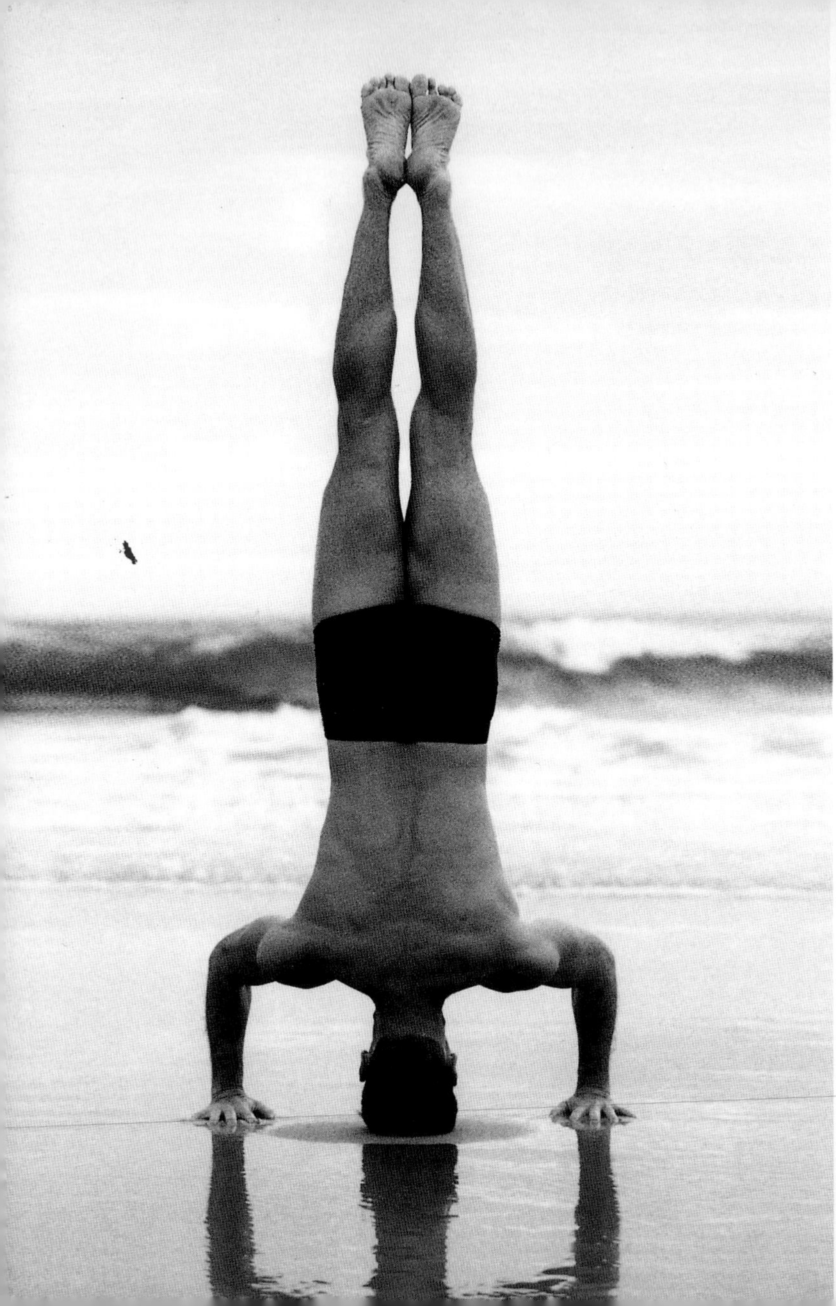

Contents

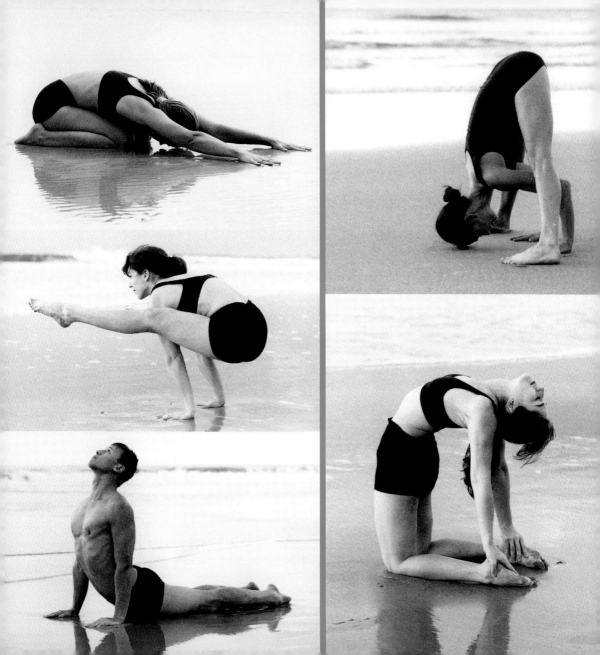

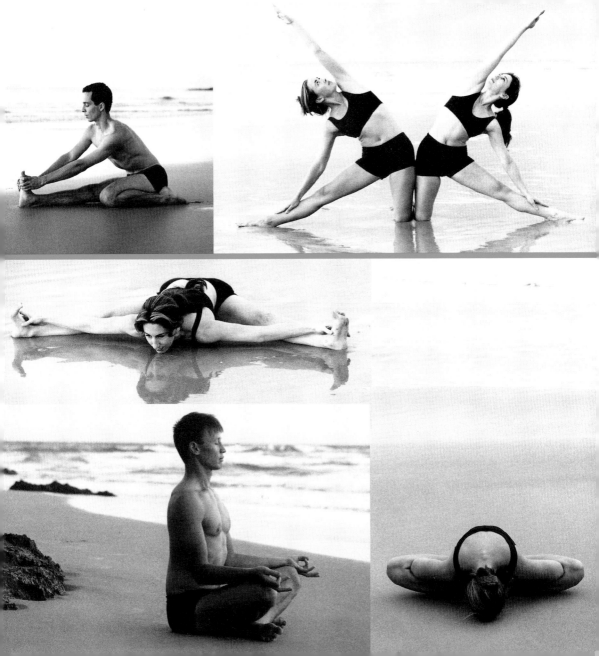

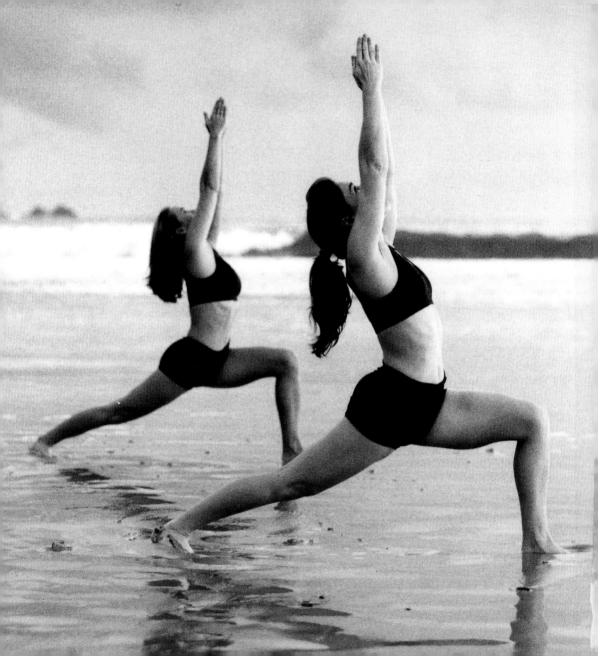

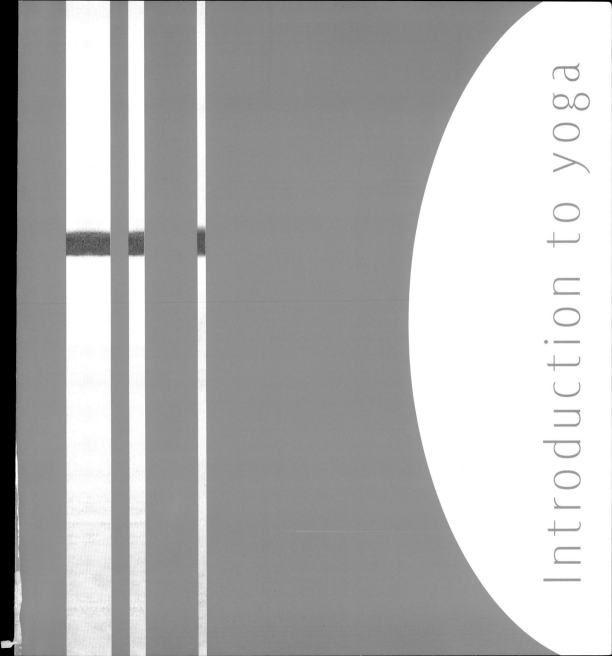

Introduction to yoga

What is yoga?

The word yoga symbolises the union of oneself with all that is.

Through the practice of yoga we experience increased self-awareness and feelings of centredness, clarity and balance in our everyday lives. We are more able to make important choices necessary in realising our potential. Yoga is an internal practice that is unique to each individual. Whether you first come to it through the postures, the philosophy or through meditation, you will be enriched with personal insights and revelations.

Yoga aims to balance all the aspects of the self: physical, emotional, mental and spiritual and to bring out the best in each individual. It offers us a way to live a healthy and harmonious life. The mental and physical disciplines taught in yoga are tools for overcoming the limitations we place on ourselves, such as unhealthy lifestyle habits and mental or physical imbalances.

Yoga is a spiritual practice. It teaches us to journey within, to get to know ourselves and, ultimately, to live in harmony with our soul and the 'universal soul' or 'god'.

Yoga through the ages

Yoga has been practised and passed on for thousands of years. Originating in India, the first references to yoga, its philosophy and its many postures were discovered in some of the oldest written manuscripts ever found.

In ancient India scriptures were written in Sanskrit, a sacred language spoken and understood only by the educated and privileged few. For hundreds of years yoga remained inaccessible to the masses because of this language barrier. However, as interest in yoga grew, its philosophy became more refined and more widely understood.

A lot of what is known of yoga today is due to the collected works and translations of Patanjali – an Indian sage and yogi from around 300 BC. Patanjali wrote what are known as the *yoga sutras*. These *sutras* are short teachings offering wisdom and insights into yoga philosophy. They were easily grasped and passed down by word of mouth by those yoga students who could not read or write.

With the dedicated study and practice of yoga teachers and practitioners throughout India, yoga soon spread to other parts of the world. Today there are many styles of yoga available, each with its own emphasis. However, the teachings and the essence of yoga remain the same throughout time.

The eightfold path

In the *yoga sutras* Patanjali set down the eightfold path to the strengthening and evolution of the body, mind and soul. This eightfold path is made up of mental and physical disciplines.

Patanjali referred to each discipline as a 'limb'. Each limb develops with practice and is connected to the seven other limbs. The eightfold path is not a step-by-step manual to enlightenment – different aspects of the path may unfold at different stages in our lives.

The eightfold path helped illuminate the philosophy behind yoga, making yoga more accessible to the spiritual seeker.

The eight limbs of yoga

1.) YAMA

These are five universal ethics that act as a guide for us to live in harmony with one another in a shared and peaceful world.

Ahimsa – non-violence, physical or otherwise

Satya – truthfulness to oneself and to others

Asteya – non-stealing

Brahmacharya – chastity. This does not necessarily refer to celibacy, rather to the containing and harnessing of one's sexual energy for other purposes.

Aparigraha – non-hoarding or avoiding over-consumption

2.) NIYAMA

These are five personal disciplines that relate to the body and mind. As you practise yoga, you will naturally begin to tune into these disciplines.

Saucha – purity and cleanliness. This can refer to the body, mind and environment.

Santosa – contentment. With contentment comes happiness in the moment, rather than looking to the past or future.

Tapas – devotion and dedication. This could refer to a teacher, spiritual path, or any topic of interest. *Tapas* encourages inspiration and personal growth.

Svadhyana – study, observation and awareness of the self.

Isvara Pranidhana – devotion to 'god' or the 'universal one'.

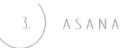

3.   A S A N A

These are the physical postures that aim to develop a healthy body and mind. Yoga *asanas* stretch and strengthen the body and release unwanted toxins. As the body grows stronger, so does your mind and willpower, preparing you for sitting quietly in meditation.

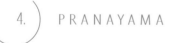

4.   P R A N A Y A M A

These are the techniques for correct breathing. Through increasing our intake of *prana*, or life force, and learning to breathe fully, our energy levels increase and our life is enriched.

5. PRATYAHARA

This is the withdrawal from the search for constant stimulation and satisfaction in the world, turning the focus inward to experience happiness from within.

6. DHARANA

This is the practice of concentration that leads to calming the mind. Entering into a quiet, meditative space becomes more effortless and more desirable.

7. DHYANA

Dhyana is meditation. Through this practice we experience the mind emptying itself of thoughts and desires and the whole being benefits from this 'time out'.

8. SAMADHI

This is the experience known as 'enlightenment', where you live completely in the moment, in union with all around you. It is the ultimate goal of yoga practice.

A s a n a

Asana means posture. It is the third limb on the eightfold path with the aim of developing a healthy body and mind to live a full and balanced life. The body is stretched and loosened, strengthened and cleansed.

The *asanas* were designed to help individuals maintain a healthy body and to prepare it for breathing exercises and sitting quietly in meditation. After a session of postures, the body is more flexible and the mind is clear and quiet. Slipping into a meditative space comes more naturally.

Yoga *asana* classes are popular all around the world. Many people choose yoga over other forms of physical exercise because of the calming and clarifying effect it also has on the mind. Not only do the postures help tone and cleanse all the systems of the body, but your sense of mental and emotional well-being greatly improves. You begin to feel your quality of life improving on all levels.

This book is a guide to inspire the beginner to yoga practice. It presents a broad range of classic yoga postures developed by experienced yoga teachers that are safe and effective for beginners. The more advanced postures which have no practical instructions are purely inspirational and are not meant to be practised from this book.

As a general guide, start with standing postures to warm up and strengthen the body. Continue with sitting and twisting postures to stretch the body more deeply. Then use a backbend, counterbalanced with a forward stretch. Wind down the practice with an inverted posture and some quiet sitting and breathing. Always end the session with a version of *Savasana*, or another relaxation postures.

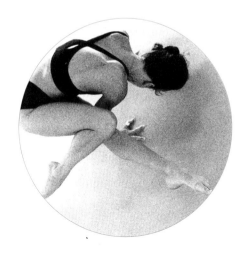

Getting to know the postures

Your energy levels vary from one day to the next and so may your enthusiasm for particular postures! Some days you might feel tired and emotional; other days on top of the world with abundant energy to spare.

Your body may go through many changes as you encourage it to open and strengthen in places you may never have been in touch with before. You will soon discover the areas of your body that are strong or weak, soft or tight. Do not strain or force your body into a posture. Let your body be in the pose and soften with the breath; your muscles will slowly become more supple.

Get to know the postures. With regular practice, the body becomes stronger and more flexible and the joints loosen. You may start out by trying only a couple of postures a day, building up your practice over time. As your awareness of the postures grows, so will your body's natural ability to perform them.

This is yoga, the body and mind working in unison.

Yoga through the day

Traditionally, yoga is practised before or at sunrise when the atmosphere is still and the mind is peaceful. However, yoga can be practised at any time of the day. Experiment with your yoga and get to know your body and how it changes throughout the day.

Yoga practised in the morning gives you lots of energy to enjoy all the day has to offer. Your body may be quite stiff after sleeping all night, so warming up slowly is important. The greeting the day sequence (page 138) warms up the body quickly and is a good way to begin any practice.

Practising yoga in the afternoon is a different experience altogether. Your body is already warmed up and you may find you have a lot less resistance to a posture you found difficult in the morning. Choose postures that will help you achieve a specific effect. Relaxation postures can help you wind down at the end of a day and calm a busy mind, or more dynamic postures can help restore much needed vitality and energy.

Evening yoga is a beautiful way to complete the day. Simply sitting quietly and concentrating on deep, full breathing is a perfect way to prepare the mind and body for a restful sleep.

Sacred space

It is best to practise yoga in a clean, quiet, dry environment free from the distractions of telephones, people and loud noises. However, if you have to make a choice between practising with your children at home or not practising at all, then of course, go ahead and practise. The kids might even get inspired to join in!

To create a sacred space for yoga if you are not part of a class you just need a little imagination. Try setting up a spare room as an inner sanctuary. Alternatively, just lighting a candle on your bedroom floor is enough to create a peaceful atmosphere. You can practise in a completely empty space, symbolic of an empty, open mind, or you can make the space special with flowers, peaceful pictures and essential oils or incense.

Varying your practice environment can also be exciting. Practising out in the fresh air is a good way to connect with nature. Find a beautiful setting that is tranquil and clean. An early morning stretch on the beach followed by a quick dip is great, as is a peaceful spot among birds in a garden.

Clothing and equipment

The beauty of yoga is that the only equipment you need is the ground you stand on – and it's free! However, as the ground is sometimes cold or uneven, it is preferable to use a rug or mat on a flat surface. Thin rubber yoga mats are helpful so you don't slip around, and they are a neat package if you are travelling and want to be sure you have your yoga 'space' wherever you go.

Yoga is usually best practised barefoot and it is preferable to wear natural fibres that allow the skin to breathe. So wear loose, comfortable clothes that don't constrict your circulation. The body cools down in relaxation and you want to be sure you don't feel cold while you are lying down. Have a long-sleeved top, a blanket and maybe some socks handy to put on when you begin relaxation. An eye bag is also good for relaxation because it not only blocks out the light but its weight calms the nerves and muscles around the eyelids for deeper relaxation.

The other props you may need can be adapted from household items. Blocks are helpful for the standing postures. If you can't reach the floor you can place a hand on a block, or a pile of books. Straps, or a piece of strong fabric, are helpful in forward bends if you can't reach your toes. A bolster or cushion to lie over and open up the chest is good. Blankets are also useful for many sitting postures.

Commonsense rules

If you're physically or mentally exhausted, do some soft, passive poses that relax the body and rejuvenate the mind rather than tiring yourself out even more by practising dynamic standing postures.

Avoid practising stimulating postures late at night as you may find yourself so energised you can't sleep properly.

Don't practise yoga on a full stomach. Leave time after eating and drinking before practising. An empty stomach makes for a lighter practice.

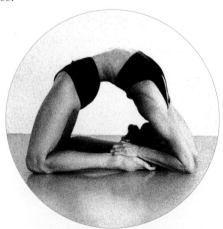

Precautions

Yoga postures have numerous benefits for the body and mind, but care should be taken when practising them. Remember that nobody knows your body better than you do, so become aware of what does and doesn't feel right. Don't push or strain yourself into a posture. If you are experiencing pain, slowly release out of the posture as you exhale.

If you know or suspect you have a medical problem, be sure to seek medical advice before practising yoga. Tell your yoga teacher about any physical problems you may be experiencing, no matter how small they may seem. An experienced teacher will be able to guide you into postures that suit your individual needs.

If you are pregnant and have never done yoga before, do not attempt any postures without first consulting your teacher. Many postures may be dangerous for the baby, but your teacher can give you safe variations. See the pregnancy sequence on page 152.

Most women experience lower energy levels when menstruating. Stick to very passive postures that keep the body cool and don't tire you out. Do not do any inverted postures. The menstruation sequence on page 146 offers relief from menstrual pain and is beneficial throughout the menstrual period.

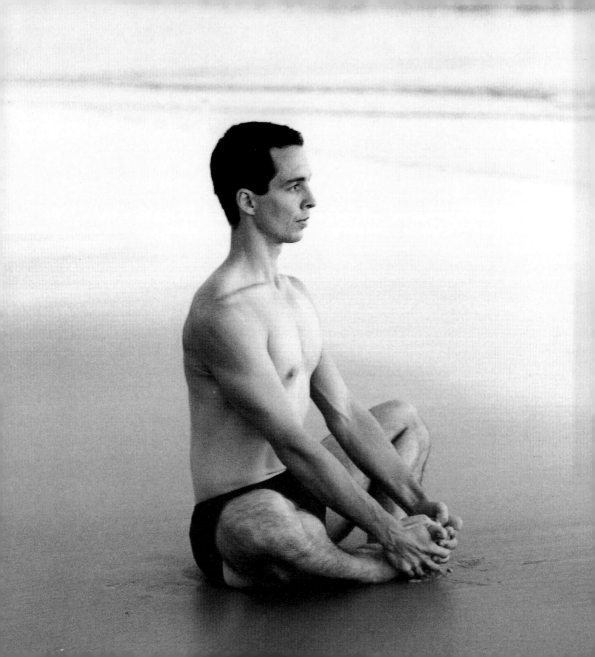

Breathing

The importance
of breathing

Learning to breathe correctly is the best health insurance you can invest in. With the world running at a faster pace than ever before, stress and anxiety are becoming the main cause of modern-day illnesses. Stress causes the chest to tighten and the breath to shorten. The systems of the body soon begin to run inefficiently.

When you breathe slowly and correctly, the muscles relax. The heart and lungs expand and the circulation of oxygenated blood throughout the body increases. When you are feeling inspired (which literally means 'to breathe in') and full of life, you can be sure that your body is receiving plenty of oxygen, particularly to the brain.

The philosophy of yoga holds that the air we breathe is full of *prana*, or life force. *Prana* is the energy that links the body with the soul, and unites our body and mind with our higher self. This *prana* gives us vitality to live a healthy and energy-filled life. Living life to our fullest potential goes hand in hand with correct breathing.

Breathing and meditation

The breath can be a focal point for meditation. When you are in a posture, observe the inhalation and exhalation of your breath. Whenever you find your thoughts wandering, return your awareness and concentration to your breath.

The mind empties of thoughts and relaxes.

After a meditative yoga practice, you will feel completely refreshed. Usually you will find any problems you were carrying before you started your practice have become more manageable. With a clear mind comes a new perspective on life.

The breath as a tool

Learn to use your breath as a tool. Developing slow, deep, rhythmic breathing allows you to move in and out of postures with ease and awareness.

When you are in a posture, use your breath to release and open tight muscles. Take your awareness to the muscles in the body that are tight or in spasm. Once you have isolated the area, take your breath there. Concentrate on letting go and softening with the exhalation. Feel the tightness melting away.

Deep, full breathing

Breathing correctly makes all the difference to our mental and emotional states. Natural breathing is slow, deep and full and indicates a relaxed state of mind. Short, tight breathing indicates a stressed and anxious body and mind.

Correct breathing is unforced, and the lungs receive maximum air. Pure, oxygenated blood circulates through the body, keeping it healthy and free of disease.

Learning to breathe correctly may require some commitment and focus but, with practice, it will become second nature. Since air is our 'food' for life, the better we breathe, the richer our life will be.

To breathe fully, first breathe in through the nose and direct the air into your abdomen. Feel your stomach expand. Then draw the air up into the lungs. The rib cage slowly expands sideways as air fills the lungs. When breathing out (through the nose), first relax your chest slightly, then your abdomen. This expels all the air from the lungs. Keep the inhalation and exhalation smooth and of equal depths.

Practise breathing correctly whenever you remember, throughout the day. With practice, natural healthy breathing will occur without you needing to focus on it consciously.

Breathing well affects your whole life. If your breathing is full and relaxed, so your life will be. Your body will function more effectively and be less prone to stress and disease. Your mind will be clearer and more focused. Your energy levels will increase, as will your inspiration and vitality.

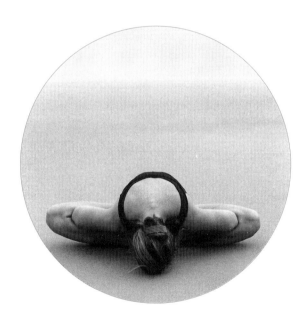

Sitting with the breath

The ancient Indian yogis believed that each individual is born with a certain number of breaths to live. They taught that the way we breathe is of vital importance to our quality and quantity of life. To slow down the breath is, in this sense, extending our lifetime. Sitting and observing the breath and increasing its length takes focus and practice. The amount of energy you have will increase dramatically, as will your vitality and enjoyment in life.

Sit in a comfortable position with your spine straight. A straight back balances the spine and allows oxygenated blood to flow easily through your body. Let your shoulders relax: down and back to open your chest, heart and lungs. Rest the backs of the hands on your knees. Relax your facial muscles as well as your head, neck and shoulders. Keeping still while you are sitting requires discipline and practice. Use the wall for support if you need to but make sure you keep your spine erect. To draw your attention inward and away from external distractions, close your eyes and focus on the inhalation and exhalation.

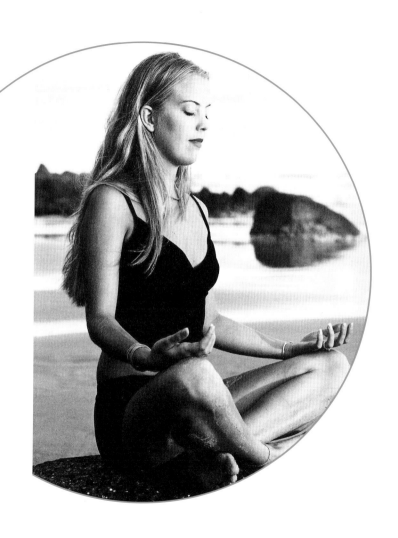

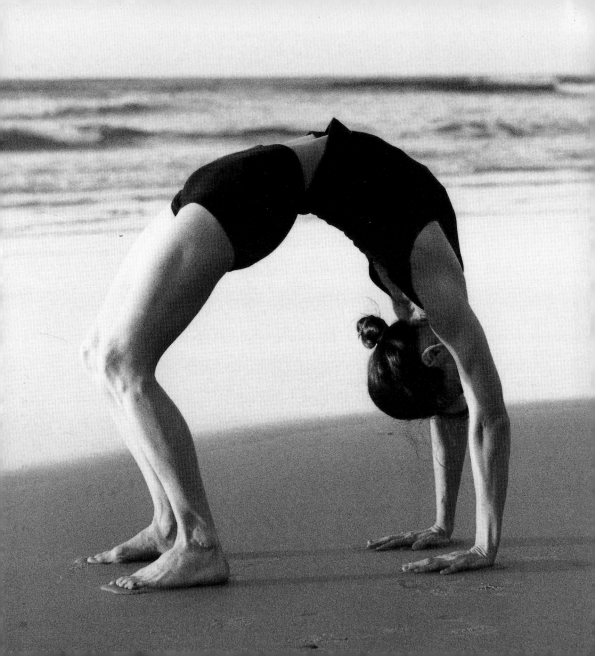

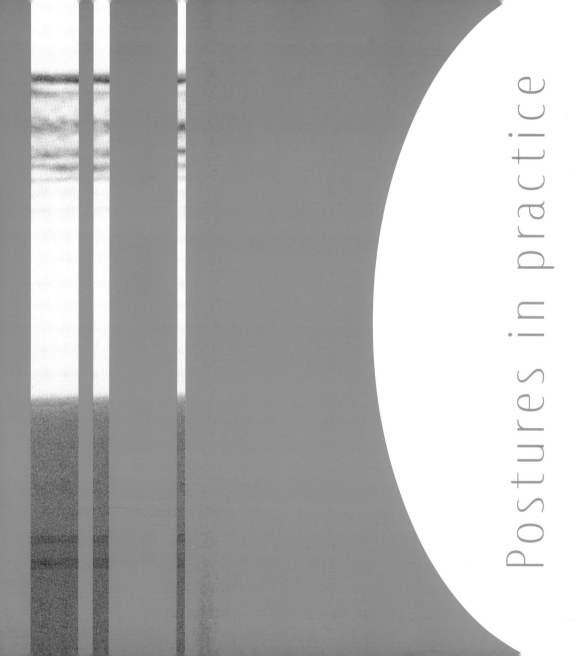

Postures in practice

Standing postures produce many physical benefits. They strengthen the body and increase flexibility. The postures flex and strengthen muscles and tendons in the legs, help to develop a supple back, and tone the spinal cord and the whole nervous system. They massage and cleanse the internal organs, and improve breathing too.

As you practise these postures, you will begin to stand, walk and sit with more awareness. You will feel as though you have grown inches taller.

Remember to check with a medical practitioner first if you suffer from any medical problems. Don't try standing postures if you suffer from high blood pressure, heart problems or nervous disorders, or if you are in the first three months of pregnancy or in the first three days of menstruation. Take extra care if you have knee or back problems.

You can avoid potential problems by becoming more aware of your body and its response to certain movements. If a posture causes pain, slowly release out of it with your breath.

Standing postures

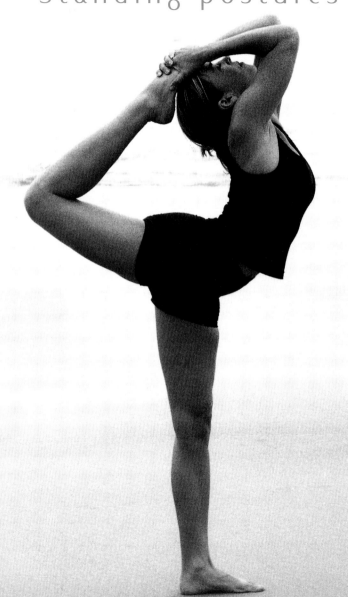

Tadasana

TADA — MOUNTAIN

Positioning: Stand with your feet together with the heels and toes touching. Bring your awareness to the soles of your feet and distribute your body weight evenly between the right and left side, back and front. Lift your calves, kneecaps and thighs up towards your hips, activating the muscles in your legs. Activate and tuck your buttocks under. Draw your abdomen in slightly. Feel your spine extending up out of your hips, and relax your shoulders down and back to open up your chest, heart and lungs. Activate your arms and extend out through your hands and fingers.

Breathing: Inhale and exhale using deep, slow breaths to expand your chest fully.

Focus: Keep the point of balance between the body and mind being relaxed as well as activated, and focus your eyes softly and directly ahead at eye level.

Hold: For ten breaths or as long as it is comfortable.

Benefits: As the vertebrae separate, the spine elongates and the spinal muscles are strengthened. This is an especially beneficial *asana* for anyone with bad posture as it aligns the skeleton correctly.

The **whole** body is filled with **energy** and **awareness**. Mind and body unite to **align** and **centre** the body's weight. Standing straight and tall, the whole body is revitalised.

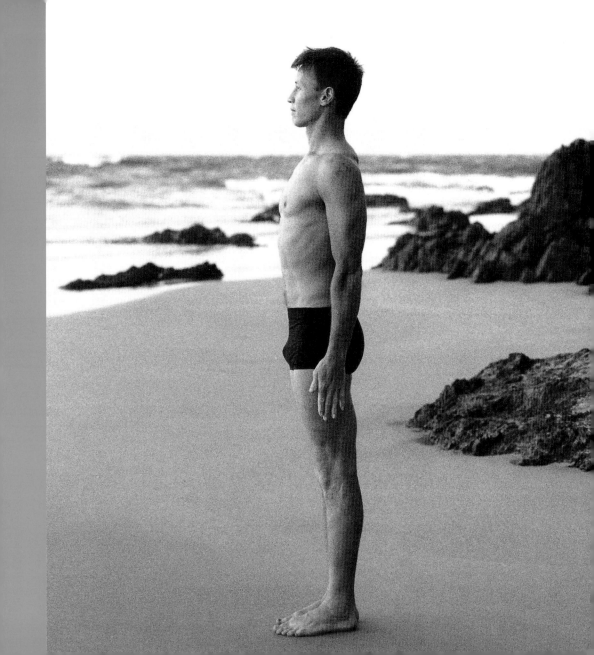

Vrksasana

VRKSA — TREE

Positioning: Stand in *Tadasana*. Bend your right leg and place the foot into your left thigh so it feels locked in. Move your right knee back to open up your hip. Keep your left leg muscles activated and lifting. Centre your body weight so you don't slant over onto your standing leg. Have your hands in prayer position in front of your heart. Drop your shoulders and roll them back. Open your chest and relax your facial muscles.

Breathing: Breathing should be deep and full, lifting and opening your rib cage up and out to the sides as you inhale.

Focus: Have your eyes gaze at a point directly in front of you, and breathe softly and evenly through your nose.

Hold: For ten breaths. Exhale to release your right leg down and repeat the posture on the other side.

Variation: Place one hand on a wall for support to maintain your balance.

Benefits: This posture teaches balance and strengthens and stretches the leg and feet muscles. It also soothes the mind and nervous system and develops concentration.

It is a great feeling to find your balance and maintain it. Once you find your balance, enter into a quiet, empty mind space free of thoughts.

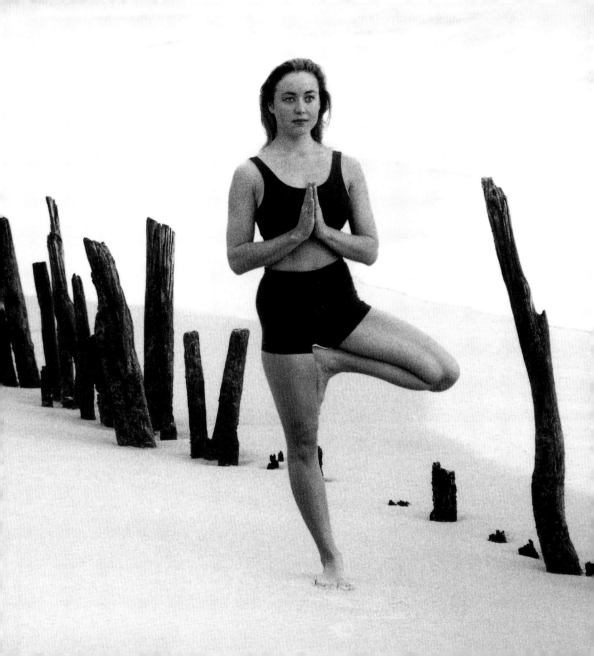

Trikonasana

TRIKONA — TRIANGLE

Positioning: From *Tadasana* place your feet 120 centimetres apart. Turn your left foot in 15 degrees and your right foot out to a 90-degree angle. Spread your toes and the base of your feet and activate your leg muscles, lifting them upwards. Extend your arms out at shoulder height. Inhale and stretch and lengthen the right arm and side of your torso over to the right, then exhale as you place your hand onto your right foot, or wherever it reaches along your leg. Extend your left arm up and tuck your chin in as you turn your head to face your left hand. Extend your arms away from each other, forming one straight line.

Breathing: Use your breath as a tool to extend and turn your left hip backwards. Inhale and exhale fully, feeling your whole body come alive.

Focus: Let your eyes focus beyond your left fingertips, slowing down your breath. Keep your body aligned and balanced.

Hold: For five breaths. Inhale to come up and out of the posture. Repeat on the other side.

Variations: Practise the posture with your back up against a wall, moving your left hip, back and shoulders toward the wall for maximum opening. If your neck becomes sore, turn your head to look down at your right foot.

Benefits: This posture stimulates and massages the nervous system, internal organs, digestive system and muscles of the spine. It also relieves tightness in the lower back and tones the lateral muscles of the torso.

The body learns coordination as it extends sideways to form a triangular shape. The whole body opens out and the muscles of the legs and torso are toned.

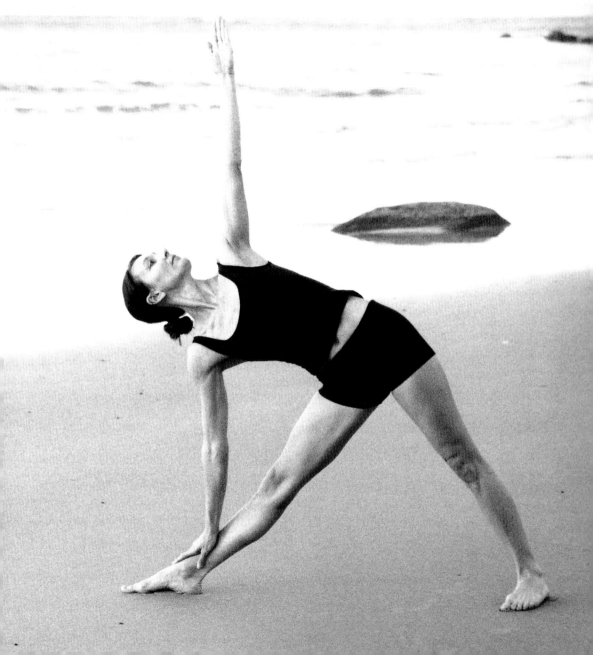

Parsvakonasana

PARSVA – SIDEWAYS; KONA – ANGLE

Positioning: From *Tadasana* place your feet 120 centimetres apart. Turn your right foot out 90 degrees and your left foot in 15 degrees. Inhale and lift out from your waist, extending your arms away from each other. Exhale as you bend your right knee into a right angle, and place your right hand on the floor on the outside of your right foot. Inhale and extend your left arm over your head, keeping your buttocks activated and your leg muscles strong. Tuck in your chin and look back toward your left hand. Extend the whole left side of your body into one straight line and stretch out from your toes through your fingertips.

Breathing: Inhale and exhale deep, full breaths.

Focus: Keep your eye gaze beyond your left fingertips. Focus on the left side of your torso turning and opening upwards, keeping both arms activated and slowing down your breathing.

Hold: For five breaths. Inhale out of the *asana* and repeat on the other side.

Variations: Place your right hand on a block if you can't reach the floor. Turn to look down at the right foot if your neck becomes sore.

Benefits: This posture stimulates the nervous system and internal organs, tones and cleanses the spinal muscles, and strengthens the legs and the muscles around the knee joint.

Precaution: Be careful if you have weak knee joints.

34

At first, there seems a lot for the body to coordinate in this posture. But with practice, your muscles will build up cellular memory to 'remember' how it's done.

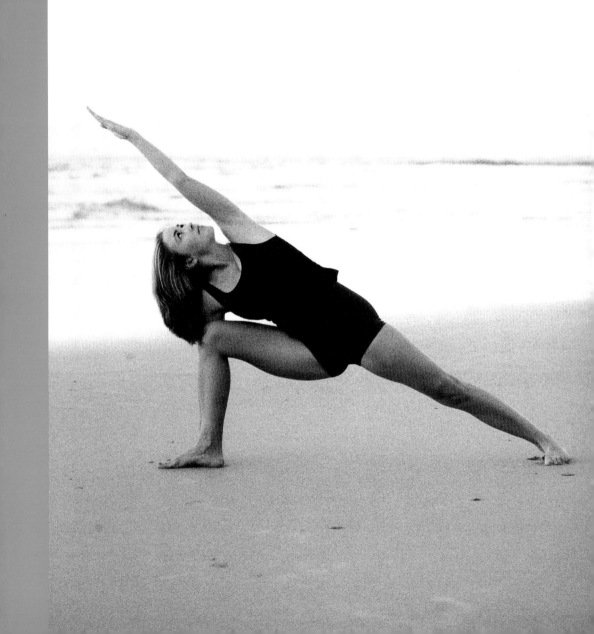

Virabhadrasana I

VIRA — WARRIOR FROM INDIAN MYTHOLOGY

Positioning: From *Tadasana* place your feet 120 centimetres apart. Turn your right foot out 90 degrees and your left foot in 45 degrees. Inhale and lift out of your waist, extending your arms upward. Turn your hips and body to the right so you are now facing the same direction as your right foot. Exhale and bend your right knee into a right angle, keeping both legs activated. Rotate your left hip forward so it is parallel to your right hip. Bring your palms together above your head and focus on your spine extending out of your hips. Look up to your hands. Feel your chest expanding with deep, full breaths. Relax your shoulders.

Breathing: Take deep, full breaths, expanding your chest fully.

Focus: Keep your eyes focused on your hands or directly ahead, and slow down your breathing.

Hold: For five breaths. Inhale to release up and out of the posture. Repeat on the other side.

Variations: If your neck becomes tired, look forward. Have your hands on your hips to avoid lower back strain or tired arms.

Benefits: This posture lengthens and tones the spinal muscles and nervous system, and strengthens the legs and the muscles of the knee joint.

In this dynamic posture the chest is puffed outwards, symbolising a warrior ready for action. The legs are the firm foundation for the extension of the upper body.

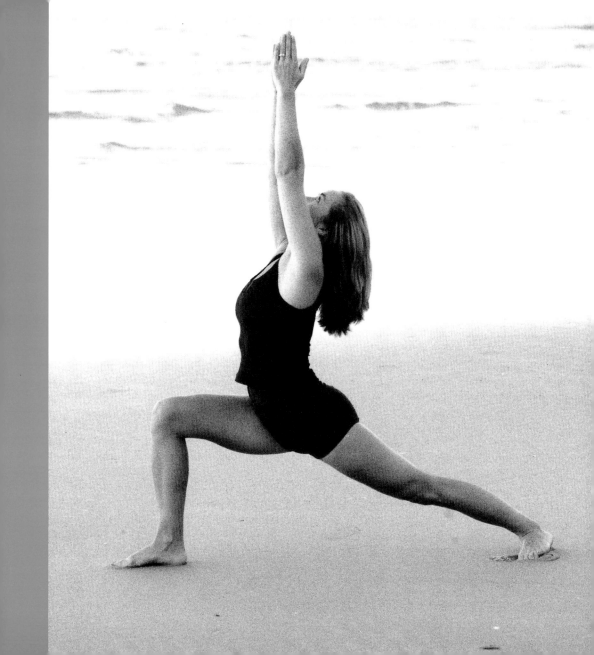

Virabhadrasana II

VIRA – WARRIOR FROM INDIAN MYTHOLOGY

Positioning: From *Tadasana* place the feet 120 centimetres apart. Turn your right foot out 90 degrees and your left foot in 15 degrees. Align the heel of your right foot with the inner arch of your left foot. As you inhale, extend your arms out to the side and lengthen out from your waist. Exhale and bend your right knee to a right angle, opening your right hip. Keep your left leg straight, with the outside of your foot touching the ground, and your buttocks activated. Lean your torso back slightly toward your left leg, so your spine sits straight up and down. Keep your arms stretching away from each other at shoulder height. Turn your head to face your right hand and relax your neck and shoulders.

Breathing: Inhale and exhale softly through your nose.

Focus: Keep your eye gaze beyond the right hand. Focus on opening your chest and hips, and on breathing slowly.

Hold: For five breaths. Inhale as you come out of the *asana* and repeat on the other side.

Variation: Perform the posture next to a wall, pressing your legs, buttocks, back and shoulders against the wall.

Benefits: This posture tones the spinal muscles and nervous system and strengthens the legs and the muscles around the knee joint.

Precaution: This is a strenuous posture, so take it easy. If your knee joints are weak, be particularly careful and stop if you feel sore.

This is another posture inspired by the mythological warrior. The body and mind are open, activated, focused and prepared for action.

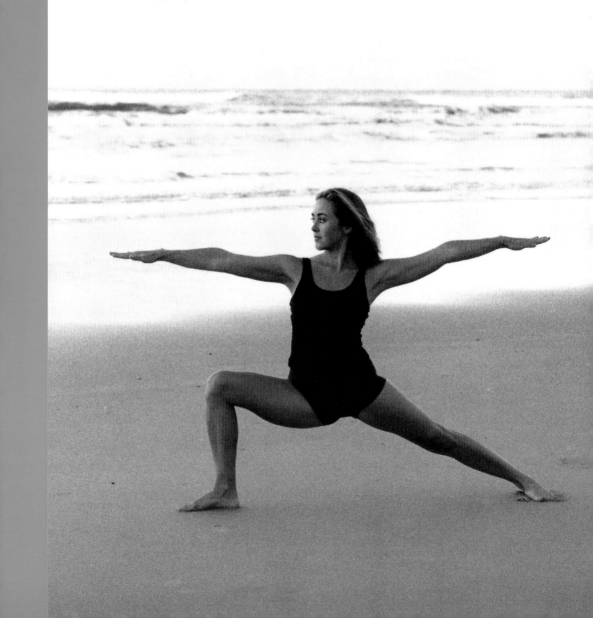

Virabhadrasana III

VIRA – WARRIOR FROM INDIAN MYTHOLOGY

Positioning: From *Tadasana* move into *Virabhadrasana I* (page 36). Exhale and extend your torso over your right leg while lifting your back leg off the ground. Extend your arms out straight, and your left leg straight out to the height of your hips. Keep your back flat and your hips parallel; the standing leg needs to be activated and firm to maintain steady balance. Extend out through your arms and fingertips and relax your facial muscles. Your arms, torso and raised leg should form one straight line.

Breathing: Breathe softly and evenly through your nose.

Focus: Keep a soft eye gaze beyond the fingertips, slowing down your breath and keeping your body balanced and in correct alignment.

Hold: For five breaths. Inhale back to *Virabhadrasana I* to release from the pose. Repeat on the other side.

Variation: Rest your hands on a bench for balance and support.

Benefits: This posture strengthens and tones the legs, arms and trunk muscles, develops willpower, and teaches the mind and body to work in unison to coordinate and balance.

In this third warrior *asana* the body forms a straight line and learns balance and coordination. The posture helps develop inner strength and focus.

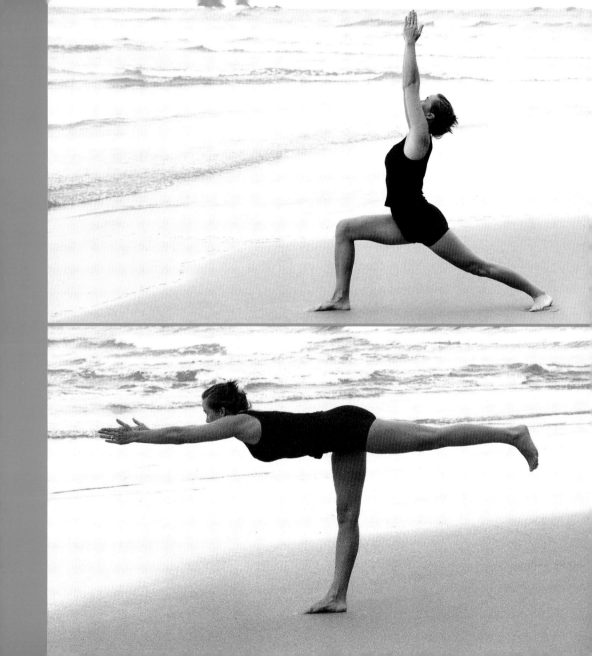

Ardha Chandrasana

ARDHA — HALF; CHANDRA — MOON

Positioning: From *Tadasana* move into *Trikonasana* (page 32). Exhale and bend your right knee as you bring your right hand to the floor in front of your foot. Straighten your right leg as you raise your left so the two legs form a right angle. Activate your buttocks, extend out of your left foot and feel the whole front of your body opening. Rotate your left hip around and back and activate the muscles of the leg you are standing on to maintain your balance. When you have your balance, raise your left arm straight up. Tuck in your chin and turn your head to look up to your hand. Feel your chest opening out.

Breathing: Breathe softly and evenly through your nose.

Focus: Keep your eye gaze beyond the left hand, opening up your left hip. Focus on finding and maintaining balance and breathing slowly.

Hold: For five breaths. To come out of the posture, inhale as you move back into *Trikonasana*, then back to *Tadasana*. Repeat the posture on the other side.

Variations: Place your right hand on a brick. Use a wall to support your back and legs and maintain balance.

Benefits: This posture strengthens the legs and buttocks and teaches focus, balance, and coordination of body and mind.

Coordinating your body into this posture requires mental and physical focus. With practice it can be accomplished gracefully.

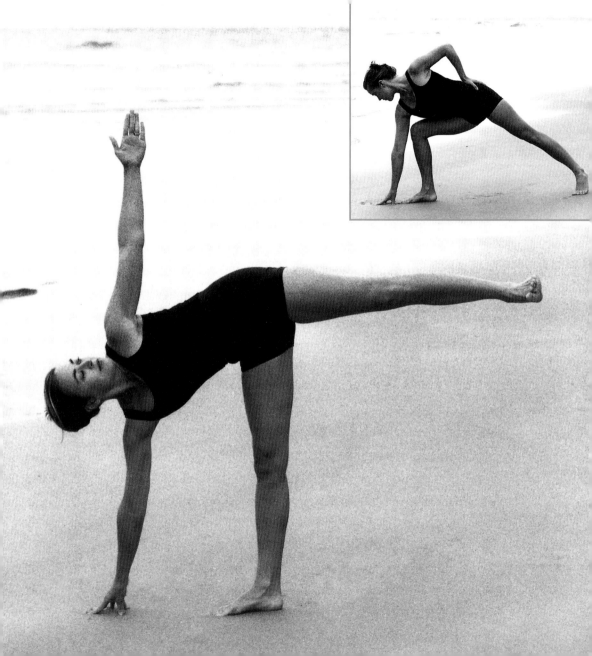

Parsvottanasana

PARSVA — SIDEWAYS; UTTAN — EXTENSION

Positioning: Place your feet 120 centimetres apart. Fold your arms behind your back with the thumbs into the crease of your elbows. Inhale and lift up out of your waist. Exhale and rotate your right foot out 90 degrees and your left foot in 60 degrees. Turn your hips and body to face the direction of your right foot. Inhale and drop your head back slightly, moving into a small back arch and opening up your chest. Exhale and extend forward to lie your torso over your right leg. If you can rest your chin on your shin, keep your leg muscles activated and rotate your right hip back and left hip forward so they are in line with each other.

Breathing: Take deep, full, even breaths, extending down a little more with each exhalation.

Focus: Keep your eye gaze toward your foot, concentrating on keeping your hips even, lengthening your spine and activating your leg muscles.

Hold: For five breaths. Release up with the inhalation. Rotate your feet and repeat on the opposite side.

Variation: Bring the palms of your hands together in a prayer position behind your back for a more intense shoulder stretch. For stability, place your hands on the floor on either side of your leg.

Benefits: This posture stretches the back muscles, massages the spinal nerves, stretches and opens the leg muscles and stimulates the intestines for good digestion.

In this *asana* the legs create a wide, triangular, stable foundation. From this the torso is free to extend and lengthen.

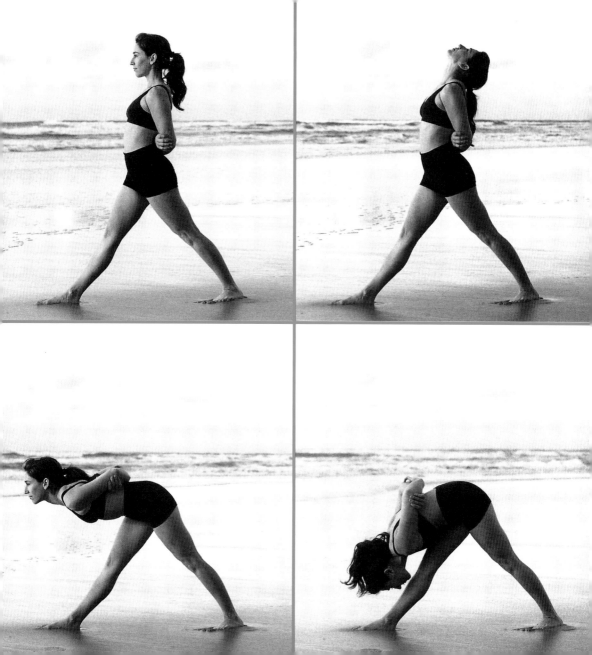

Padottanasana

PADA – FOOT/LEG; UTTAN – EXTENSION

Positioning: From *Tadasana* place your feet 150 centimetres apart. Put your hands on your hips. Inhale and extend up and out of your waist. Exhale and extend forward and halfway down so your back is flat. Slowly exhale all the way down, drawing in your torso fully toward your legs. Place the palms of your hands on the floor between your feet with your elbows bent, and hang your head down, resting the crown of your head on the floor if possible. Activate the muscles of your legs for support and stability, move your body weight forward onto the front of your feet and feel your back relax and the vertebrae separating. Lift your shoulders.

Breathing: Breathe slowly and evenly through your nose, releasing your torso forward and down with the exhalation.

Focus: Keep your eye gaze on the tip of your nose, lifting your shoulders back toward your ears, softening your back and keeping your body weight moving forward.

Hold: For five to ten breaths. Inhale to come up, bringing your hands onto your hips.

Variations: Rest your hands on a block if you cannot reach the floor. Extend your torso only halfway if you find this posture difficult.

Benefits: This posture releases tight hamstring muscles, tones the legs and buttocks and calms the mind as the head rests forward.

The legs are the support while the head, torso and arms release forward and down. Feel the opening in the leg muscles. The stretch feels great!

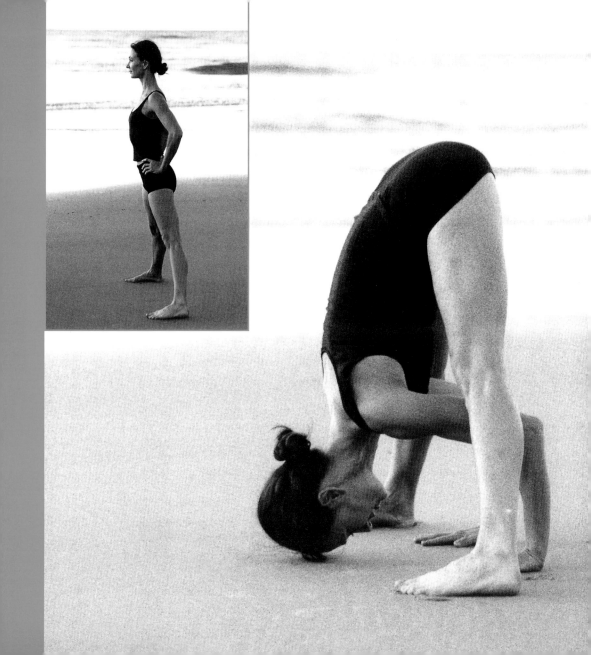

Uttanasana

UTTAN – EXTENSION

Positioning: Stand with your feet apart at hip width. Inhale and extend your arms up over your head, placing your thumbs into the crease of your elbows. Exhale and slowly release forward into the resting pose, activate your leg muscles and lock your knees. Move your body weight forward slightly onto the balls of your feet, and feel your vertebrae separating as the weight of your head, neck and shoulders draws your torso down and in toward your legs.

Breathing: Slow down your breathing and relax.

Focus: Keep your eye gaze down past the tip of your nose, or, for deep relaxation, close your eyes. Feel your spine elongating.

Hold: For ten breaths or as long as you like. Release your arms and inhale as you come up.

Variations: Bend your knees if your back feels sore. Rest the crown of your head on a cushioned chair if hanging forward is uncomfortable.

Benefits: This posture relaxes the mind, improves blood circulation and digestion, softens tight spinal muscles and reduces fat around the abdomen.

Whenever you are feeling tired or stressed, let your body and mind rest in this posture. Hanging forward quietens the mind and cools the body.

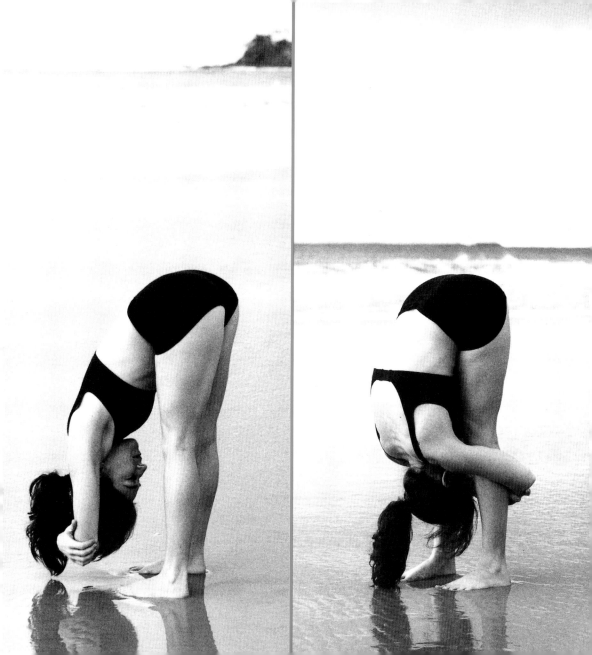

Garudasana

GARUDA — EAGLE

Positioning: Stand with the feet together in *Tadasana*. Place your hands on your hips. Bend your knees and cross your right leg over the left. If possible, tuck your right foot round and lock it behind your left ankle. Find your balance. Next, raise your bent arms to shoulder height, cross your left arm over the top of your right arm and, if possible, bring the palms together. Keep your elbows bent at a 90-degree angle and in line with your shoulders. Extend your forearms away from your head, and lift out of your waist for a spinal extension. Relax your head, neck and shoulders.

Breathing: Breathe evenly through your nose.

Focus: Find a point in front of you at eye level, and maintain your balance and stillness of mind.

Hold: For ten full breaths or as long as it is comfortable. Release and repeat the posture on the opposite side.

Variation: If it is too difficult to find your balance in this posture, practise with the hands on the hips.

Benefits: This posture strengthens and tones the muscles and nerves of the legs, loosens the joints in the legs, relieves sciatica in the legs, stretches the shoulders and teaches balance and focus.

This posture teaches balance and coordination. Once you find yourself still in the posture, your mind relaxes and the breath becomes your main point of focus.

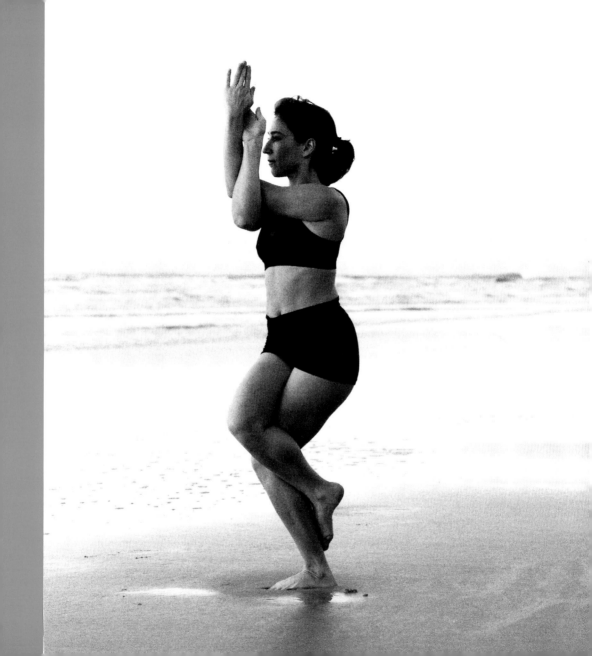

Utkatasana

UTKATA — POWERFUL

Positioning: From *Tadasana* inhale, raise your arms above your head and place the palms of your hands together. Exhale and bend your knees, keeping your heels down toward the ground. Lock your elbows, extend your spine out of your hips, lift your rib cage and breathe fully up into your chest. The torso naturally leans forward; however, try to keep your back straight and moving into an upright position. Tuck your buttocks under.

Breathing: Breathe softly through your nose.

Focus: Keep a soft eye gaze up to the hands, sitting a little lower. Keep your arms activated, flex your ankles and slow down your breathing.

Hold: For five breaths. Slowly release into a standing position as you exhale.

Benefits: This posture strengthens the back, legs, arms and torso and develops supple ankles.

This dynamic posture activates the whole body. The lower body 'sits' firmly in midair. The upper body lifts and extends.

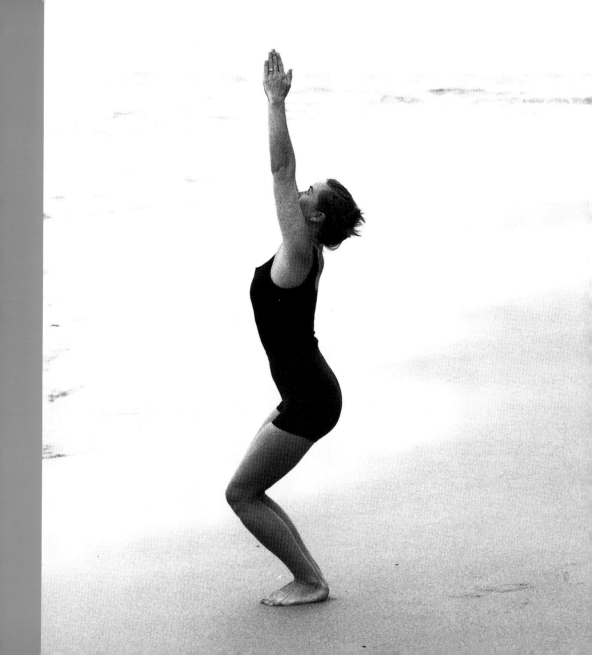

Parighasana

PARIGHA – GATE

Positioning: Kneel on the ground with your hands on your hips. Exhale and extend your right leg out to the right, keeping the foot in line with your hip. Place your right hand on your leg down toward the foot. Inhale and raise your left arm up and extend out from your waist. Exhale and extend your left arm over your head with the palm facing down. Tuck in your chin and look back toward your left hand. Feel the deep stretch in the muscles of the side of your torso and raised arm, keeping your left hip above your left knee.

Breathing: Breathe fully and use the exhalation to release further down your leg, releasing into the side stretch.

Focus: Keep your eye gaze beyond your left hand, releasing the muscles on the sides of your torso. Focus on releasing out of your hip.

Hold: For five breaths. Inhale to come up and change sides.

Benefits: This posture stretches and tones the abdomen, chest, arms and lateral torso muscles. It also stretches and softens the back muscles, massages the internal organs and tones the spinal nerves.

This intense side stretch massages and cleanses your internal organs and brings back life to the side of the torso as it stretches and opens.

54

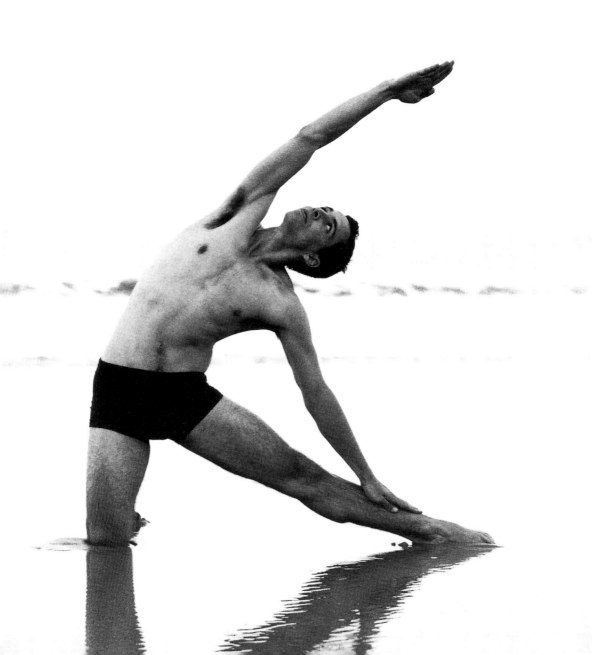

Sitting postures calm the mind and soothe the nervous system.

There are many varieties of sitting postures. Some forward-bending postures lengthen, stretch and tone the legs. Others are more focused on elongating the spine and opening up the chest and shoulders.

Because the body is resting on the floor, the sitting postures require less energy and are less strenuous than the standing postures. However, they are very effective in stretching and releasing deep into the body.

Sit on a blanket or yoga mat to cushion the body from the ground.

Stay in each posture and experience its full benefits by concentrating on your breathing while you relax and let go into the pose. Releasing muscles as you exhale is an effective, gentle and safe way to increase your flexibility.

Using a belt in some of the postures helps to extend forward and keep the hips and torso in correct alignment.

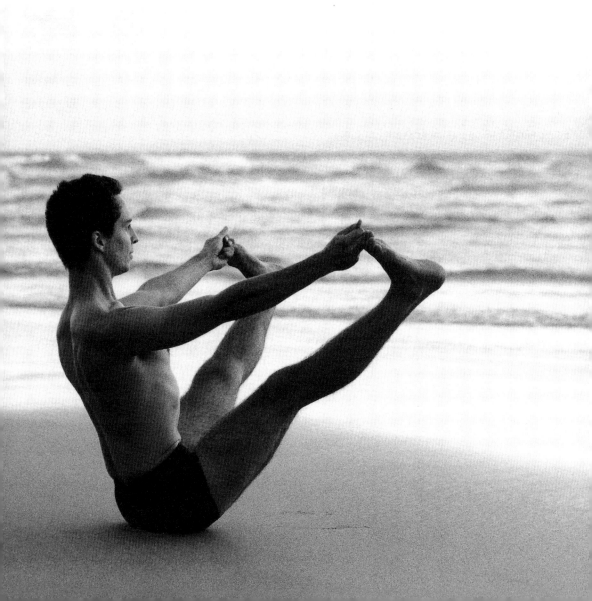

Sukhasana I

SUKHA — HAPPY

Positioning: Sit on the floor with your legs crossed. Place the back of your hands onto your knees, relax your shoulders down and roll them back to open up your chest. Focus on your spine lifting and elongating and breathe fully, expanding your chest. Keep checking to make sure your back is straight.

Breathing: This comfortable *asana* is ideal for sitting and focusing on taking deep, full, even breaths in and out through your nose.

Focus: Keep your eye gaze at a point in front or have your eyes softly closed. Focus also on keeping your back lifting, with your spine straight, as well as on opening your chest by rolling back your shoulders.

Hold: For as long as it is comfortable, then cross your legs the opposite way and repeat the posture.

Variations: Sit your buttocks on some blankets. Sit up against a wall if your back muscles are weak.

Benefits: This posture is a comfortable position to sit and practise meditation. It strengthens the spinal muscles, gently opens up the hips and stimulates blood flow to the pelvic region.

This easy cross-legged posture strengthens and straightens the back and gently opens the hips. Enjoy the calm as you sit in this centred position.

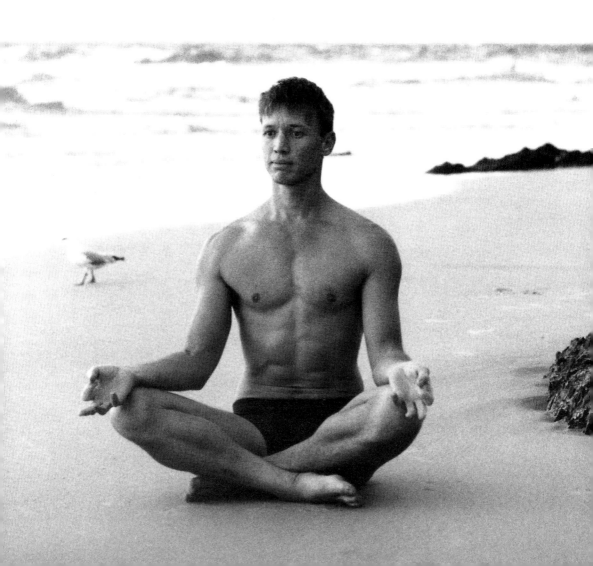

Sukhasana II

SUKHA – HAPPY

Positioning: Interlock your fingers and turn the palms outward. Raise your arms up over your head as you lift out of your waist and activate the muscle of your arms. Keep your head, neck and shoulders relaxed.

Breathing: Breathe fully and evenly as you lift and expand your chest.

Focus: Keep your eye gaze at eye level and at a point ahead. Lengthen out of your waist and keep your back straight.

Hold: For five breaths. Then interlock your fingers the opposite way and perform the posture on the other side.

Benefits: This posture separates the vertebrae, stimulates blood circulation through the spine and stretches the muscles of the sides of the torso. It gently opens the hips and stimulates blood flow to the pelvic region.

This simple upward lift brings life to the whole upper body. The extension stretches deep into the shoulder and arm muscles, releasing tightness and stress.

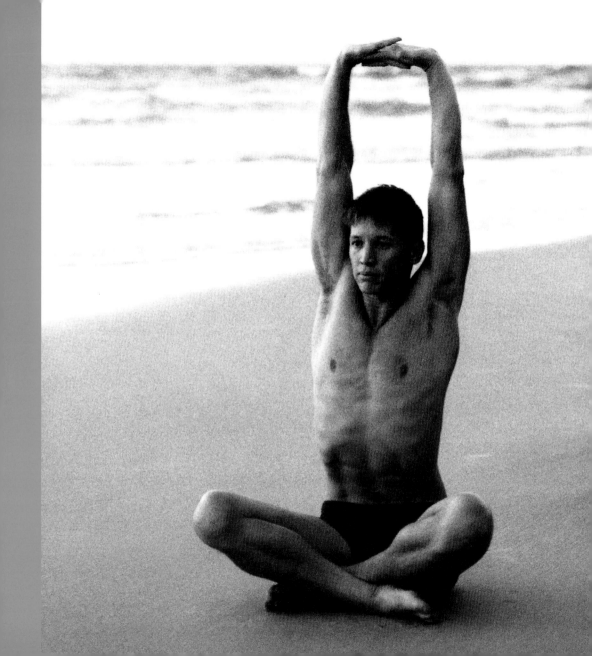

Dandasana

DANDA – STICK

Positioning: Sit with your legs stretched out and your back upright. Open up your chest by rolling your shoulders back. Feel your body correctly aligned and your weight even on your right and left buttocks. Lock your legs and arms and activate the muscles.

Breathing: Breathe fully, keeping your breath slow and even. Feel your rib cage expanding and contracting as you inhale and exhale.

Focus: Keep your eye gaze down toward your feet, and your chest and spine lifting upward. Focus also on rolling your shoulders down and back and relaxing your facial muscles.

Hold: For ten full breaths.

Benefits: This posture opens the chest, lungs and heart, teaches the spine correct posture and strengthens the muscles of the legs. The stillness of the posture quietens the mind.

The back is erect and the legs and arms are activated and straight in this posture. Become aware that the whole body is activated.

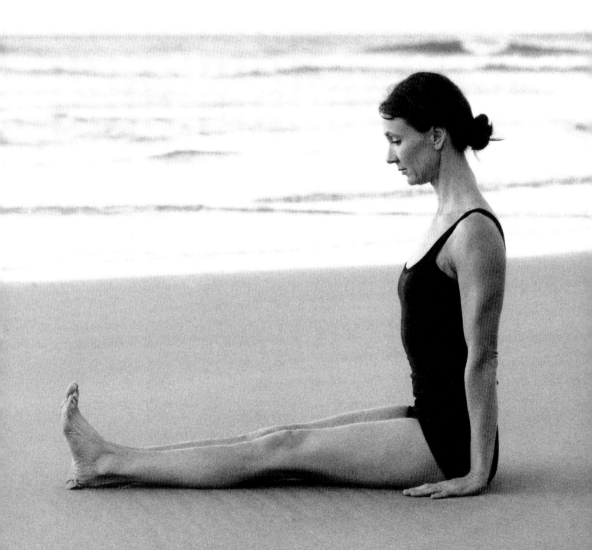

Baddha Konasana I

BADDHA — BOUND; KONA — ANGLE

Positioning: Sit with the soles of your feet together. Let your knees relax down toward the floor and the muscles around your hips soften. Interlock your fingers around your toes and lift out of your lower back. Roll your shoulders down and back, and lift and open your chest.

Breathing: Take deep, full, rhythmic breaths. Send the awareness of the exhalation to your hips, softening and letting go in the hips.

Focus: Keep your back straight and let go in your hips.

Hold: For ten breaths or as long as it is comfortable.

Benefits: This posture soothes the sacral nerves, strengthens the back muscles, releases tension in the hips and stimulates circulation to the pelvic region and reproductive organs.

This posture increases circulation to the pelvic organs. It soothes menstrual pain and helps maintain healthy reproductive organs.

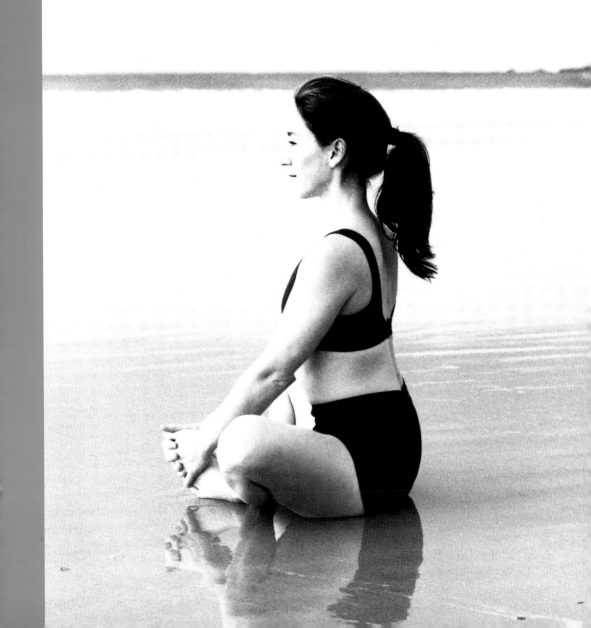

Baddha Konasana II

BADDHA — BOUND; KONA — ANGLE

Positioning: Lifting from the front of your body, stretch your torso up and bend forward and down toward the ground. Aim for your abdomen to rest along the floor, then your chest, then your chin. To open your hips further, place your elbows on your knees, working them to the floor.

Breathing: Get in touch with your breath. With a deep exhalation, relax and let go in your hips.

Focus: Feel your hips softening and opening, relax your head downward and calm your mind.

Hold: For five to ten breaths.

Variation: Rest your head on a bolster or a pile of pillows.

Benefits: These are the same as for *Baddha Konasana I*, only a little more intense. Resting your head forward and down relaxes the mind.

This forward-extending posture opens deep into the hips, releasing stiffness and stimulating blood flow to the pelvic organs.

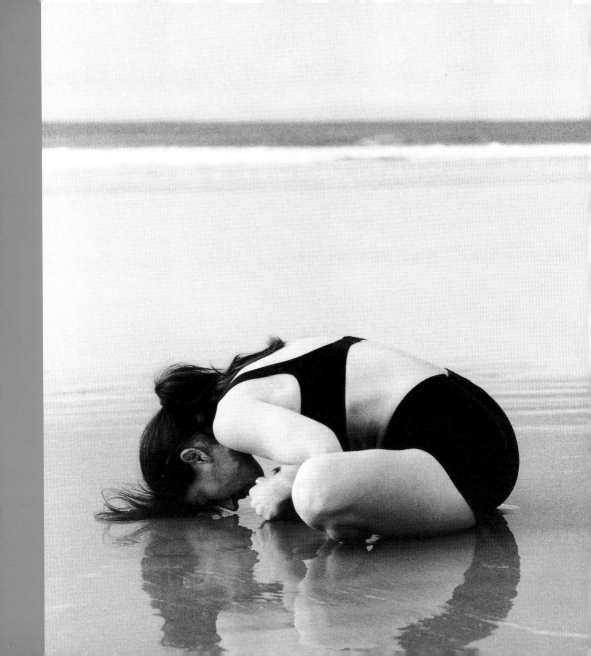

Janu Sirsasana

JANU — KNEE; SIRSA — HEAD

Positioning: Sit with your legs stretched in front of your body. Bend your right leg and place the heel of the foot into your groin. Open up the sole of your foot to face upward and feel your right hip opening. To come forward, inhale and lift out from your waist, lengthening from the front of your body. Either hold onto your feet or a belt looped around the feet and, with the exhalation, extend over your outstretched leg. Rotate your abdomen to the left so your torso is lying straight along your outstretched leg. Rest your abdomen, chest and head comfortably onto your leg.

Breathing: Breathe slowly, releasing your torso forward and down a little more each time you exhale.

Focus: Turn your eye gaze toward your foot. Focus on relaxing your back muscles and abdomen.

Hold: For five breaths. Inhale out of the posture and change sides.

Variations: Place a blanket under the knee of your outstretched leg to relieve tight leg muscles. Stay with your back upright and hold onto a belt looped around your feet if extending forward is painful. Place a bolster on your knees and rest the forehead onto it if lying forward is difficult.

Benefits: This posture stimulates blood flow to the internal organs. It tones the abdominal and leg muscles and loosens the hips.

Precautions: Do not practise this posture if you have chronic arthritis, sciatica or a slipped disc.

Your head lies forward in this position, calming the mind and cooling the whole body. Empty your mind of thoughts by focusing on the soft sound of your breath.

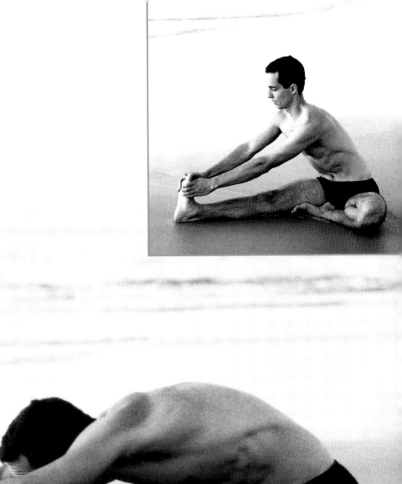
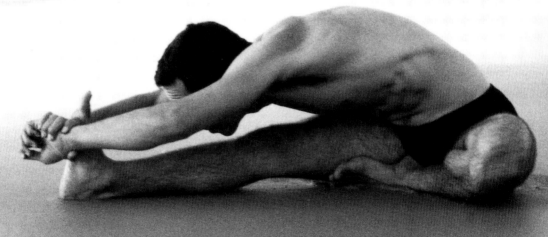

Triang Mukhaikapada Pascimottanasana

TRI – ANGLE; MUKHA – FACE; PADA – FOOT;
PASCIMOTTASANA – POSTERIOR EXTENSION

Positioning: Start with both legs stretched out in *Dandasana*. Bend your right leg back. Place a pile of blankets under your left buttock if you need support. Keep your knees pressing together. Roll your right calf muscle out. Have the sole of your right foot facing upward and the heel touching the hip. Once you are comfortable, extend up out of your waist while inhaling. Extend your arms and torso forward as you exhale. Hold onto your feet as you lie your head down onto your leg.

Breathing: Breathe deeply and slowly, lifting your chest forward with the inhalation and releasing down with the exhalation.

Focus: Send your eye gaze toward your foot, relaxing your head and neck, elongating your spine and quietening your mind.

Hold: For five breaths. Inhale out of the *asana* and repeat on the other side.

Variations: Place a blanket under the knee of the extended leg. Stay with your back upright, holding onto a belt looped around your feet if extending forward is painful. Alternatively, rest the forehead down on a bolster.

Benefits: This position stimulates blood flow to the internal organs and nervous system as well as toning the abdominal and leg muscles.

Precaution: Be careful if you have weak knees.

Keeping the body weight evenly distributed between both hips is a challenge in this posture. Take your awareness inward as you concentrate.

70

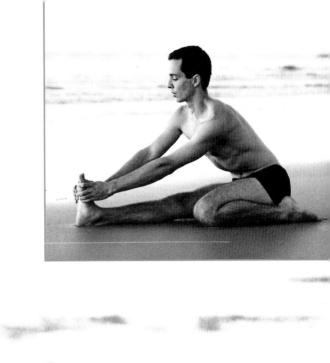

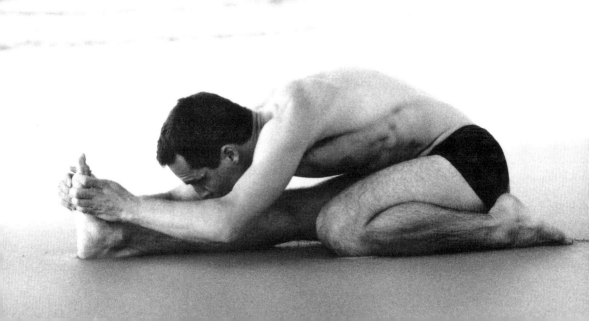

Virasana I

VIRA — A HERO

Positioning: Sit your buttocks on your heels. Slide your heels out to the side so that your buttocks release onto the ground and sit between your heels on the floor. At this point, decide whether you will need to sit on some blankets to relieve pain in your legs, knees and ankles. Draw your knees in toward each other. Stretch the sides of your torso up. Roll back your shoulders and open your chest. Rest the backs of your hands on your knees.

Breathing: Breathe evenly in and out through your nose.

Focus: Use a soft eye gaze at a point ahead, keeping your back straight and the bones of your buttocks down.

Hold: For as long as it is comfortable.

Variations: Kneel with your legs on a pile of blankets to relieve tight ankles and feet. Sit your buttocks on a pile of blankets to release strain in your legs.

Benefits: This posture activates the digestive system and is good for relieving indigestion if practised after a heavy meal. It strengthens pelvic muscles, knee and ankle joints, stimulates blood flow to the pelvic organs and is a good posture for meditation if the body is comfortable staying in it.

Practise this posture to open up tight knees and ankles. Once you can sit in it comfortably it becomes a soothing, resting pose for any time of day.

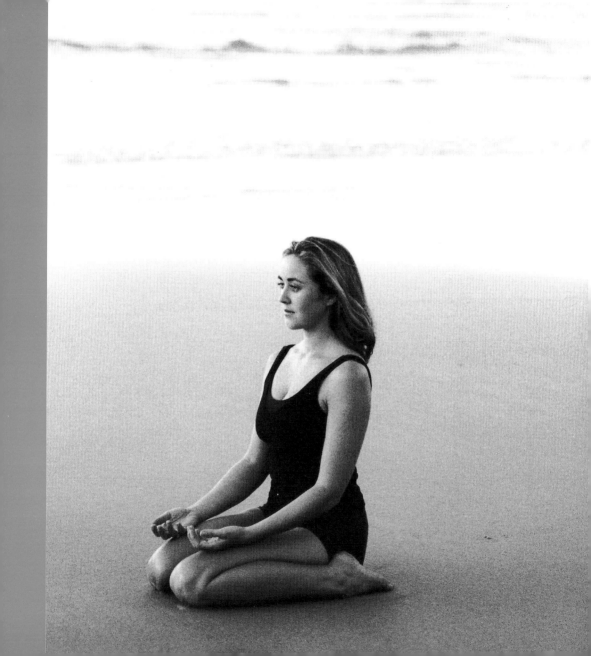

Virasana II

VIRA — A HERO

Positioning: Sit in *Virasana I*. Inhale and raise the arms above the head. Exhale, bend and extend the torso and arms forward and down. Rest the forehead on the floor. Keep the buttocks back to the heels.

Breathing: Maintain natural breathing, softening into the pose with the exhalation.

Focus: Keep the focus on the breathing. Close your eyes and sink your forehead to the floor.

Hold: For five breaths. Exhale when you release up.

Benefits: This posture tones the muscles of the pelvis and stimulates blood flow to the pelvic organs, which helps to maintain healthy functioning of the reproductive organs. It also helps relieve sciatica.

This forward-extension posture stretches deep into the ankle and knee joints, opening and releasing tightness. The spine extends and gently stretches.

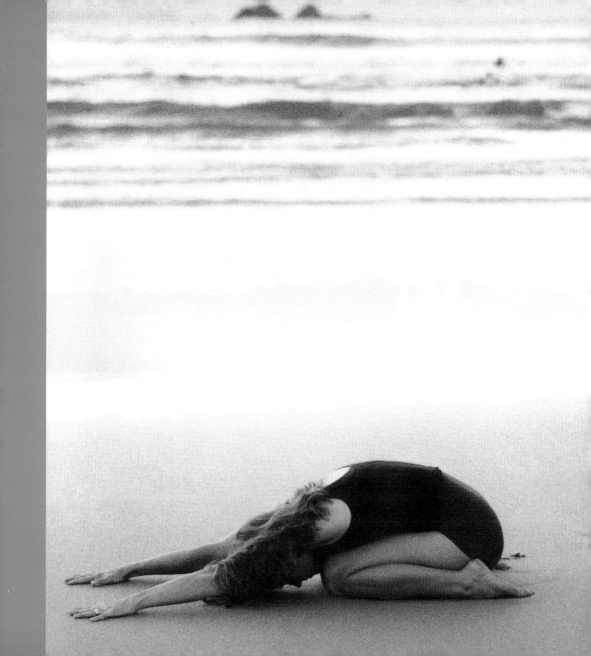

Parvatasana

PARVA — MOUNTAIN

Positioning: Sit in a comfortable cross-legged position. Inhale and raise your arms, placing the palms together above your head. Bend your elbows slightly. Relax your shoulders down and open your chest.

Breathing: Inhale and exhale in slow, even breaths.

Focus: Keep a soft eye gaze at a point in front or have your eyes softly closed, keeping your arm muscles activated and lifting and focusing inward on a quiet space empty of thoughts.

Hold: For five to ten breaths. Exhale to release your arms down and repeat the posture with your legs crossed the other way.

Benefits: This posture strengthens the arms, lengthens the spine and softens the hip muscles. It develops willpower and quietens the mind.

With the hands raised in prayer position, this is a beautiful posture that invokes a quiet and meditative space.

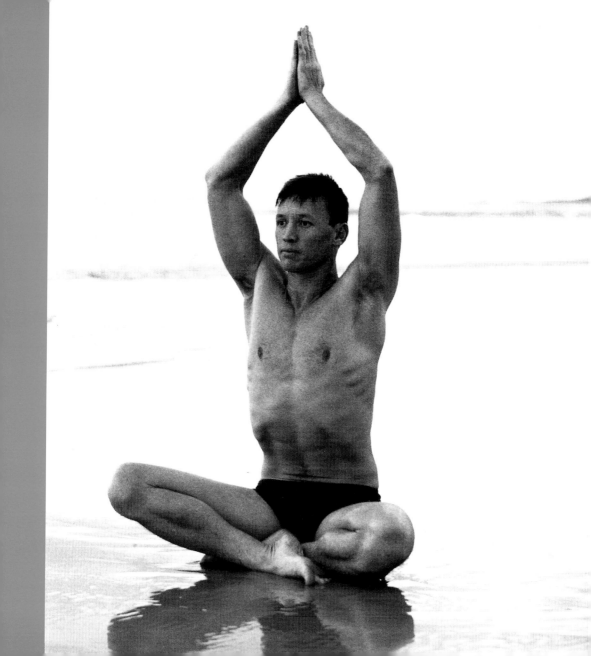

Navasana

NAU – BOAT

Positioning: Find your balance on the front of your sitting bones. Raise your legs halfway in towards your chest and extend your arms out parallel to them. Move around until you feel you are centred. Lift your lower back in and up so it doesn't collapse.

Breathing: Inhale to raise your body. Breathe slowly and evenly while you are in the posture. Exhale to release your body.

Focus: Extend your eye gaze beyond the feet, pulling your back in and up and activating your stomach, leg and arm muscles.

Hold: For five to ten full breaths.

Variation: For a more intense pose, raise and straighten your legs and lock your knees. The arms stay parallel to the floor. Your torso and legs will form a 'V' shape.

Benefits: This posture stimulates digestion and strengthens the abdominal muscles as well as the back, legs and arms.

This posture teaches alignment, balance, centring, and focus. With practice, you will appreciate the feeling of lightness that comes with Navasana.

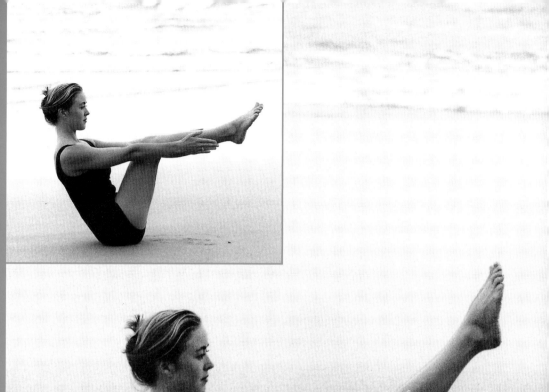
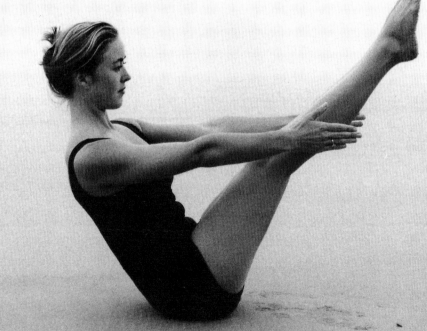

Twists are powerful postures that help maintain a clean and healthy body. Twists soften tight back muscles, release toxins and improve the circulation of blood and oxygen through the spine. The internal organs are massaged and the intestines are stimulated to promote good digestion and bowel function. If you spend a lot of time sitting at a desk, a regular spinal twist will help relieve a tired, sore back.

These postures should be practised carefully. Use exhalations to soften and release deeper into a twist. Twist to both sides of the torso for equal lengths of time and rest after twisting.

When releasing from a spinal twist you may feel a rush of energy. Often the twist affects the body so powerfully that the release of toxins and blocked energy is immediate.

If you suffer from any spinal problems, seek medical advice before attempting the twisting *asanas*. Do not attempt the twisting postures if you are pregnant.

Twisting postures

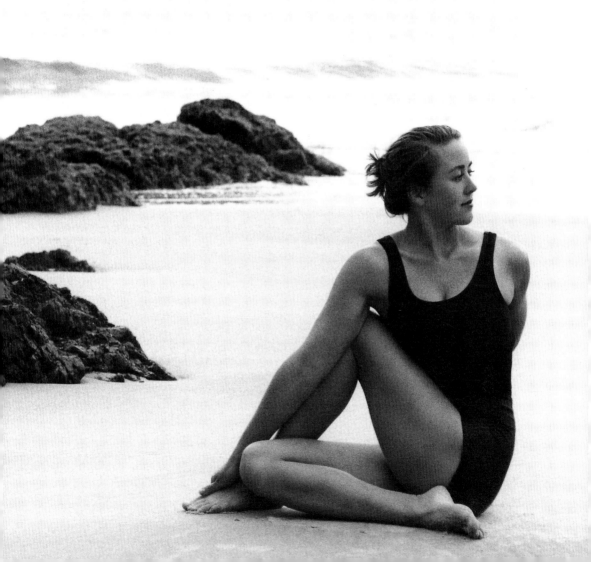

Bharadvajasana

BHARADVAJA — AN INDIAN SAGE

Positioning: Sit on your buttocks with your legs bent sideways to sit beside your left hip. Place your right foot underneath your left foot. Inhale up out of your waist and twist your torso and head to the right. Place your left hand beside your right knee and your right hand on the ground behind your right hip. Inhale and raise your right arm and wrap it around your back to hold onto your left elbow. Rotate your right shoulder and elbow back, and turn your head to look over your left shoulder.

Breathing: Breathe slowly and evenly. Bring your awareness to the point where the spine is twisting and release deeper into the twist with your breath.

Focus: Keep your eye gaze beyond your left shoulder, and lift and open your chest.

Hold: For five breaths or as long as it is comfortable. Practise the posture on both sides.

Benefits: This posture tones the spinal muscles and nervous system and relieves tight shoulders or a stiff back.

This simple, effective posture relieves backache. The twisting action softens tight muscles, releasing tension and stimulating blood flow through the spine.

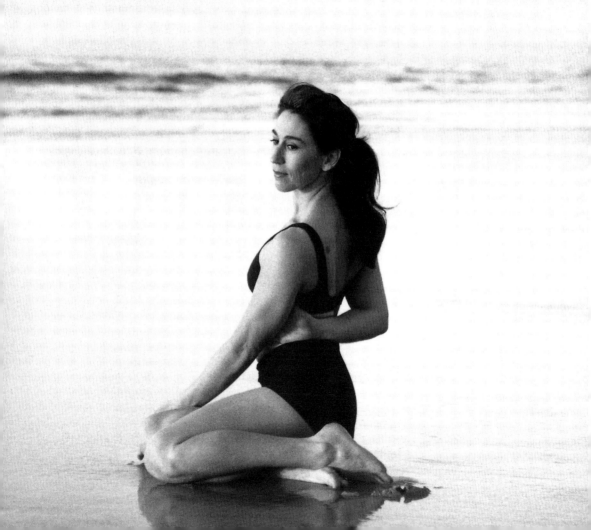

Maricyasana Twist

MARICI – AN INDIAN SAGE

Positioning: Sit on the ground with your legs stretched out. Bend your right leg and place the foot close up to the groin, so your thigh touches your abdomen. Inhale and turn to place your right hand on the ground behind your right hip. Lock your left arm in front of your right knee, pressing your knee into your arm. Inhale and lift out of your hips, thinning your waist. Exhale and turn to look back over your right shoulder. Keep your left leg straight and the muscles activated.

Breathing: Use the breath as a tool to lift and turn into the twist. As you inhale, lift your spine. As you exhale, turn and twist your spine and spinal muscles.

Focus: Keep your eye gaze beyond your right shoulder, and your bent knee upright.

Hold: For five breaths. Release your arms and repeat on the other side.

Benefits: This posture stretches and tones the spinal cord, relieves backache, rejuvenates the brain and gives the internal organs a cleansing massage.

This twisting posture gives an internal massage to the body's systems. It cleanses sluggish internal organs and releases toxins.

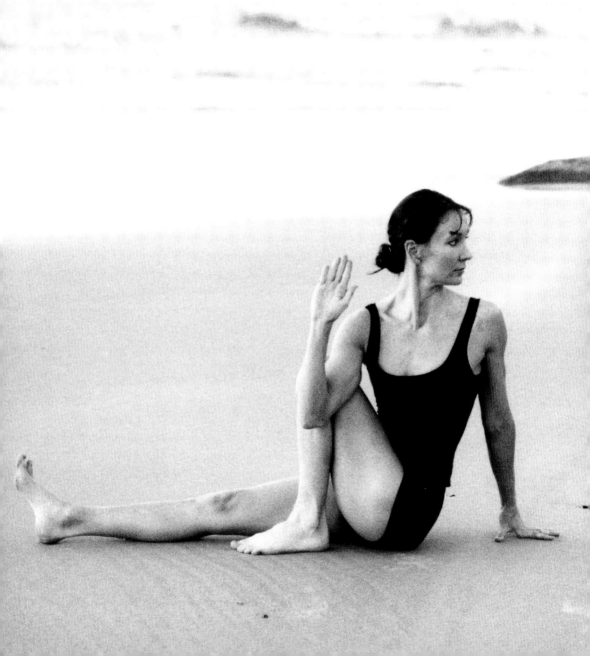

Spinal Roll

Positioning: Lie flat on the ground with your legs straight. Extend your arms out to the side with the palms facing down. Inhale and bend your knees into your chest. Exhale and turn your head to face down beyond your left hand. Exhale and release the bent legs down to the right onto the ground. Place your knees in close to your right armpit. Keep both shoulders flat to the floor.

Breathing: Breathe deeply.

Focus: Keep your eye gaze beyond your left hand. Focus on softening the back and keeping your shoulders to the ground.

Hold: For five breaths. Inhale, raise your legs back to the centre and change sides.

Benefits: This posture tones the spinal cord, stretches back muscles and releases tension in the upper back.

The muscles supporting the spine can easily become tired and inflexible. This simple twist keeps your back soft, supple and healthy.

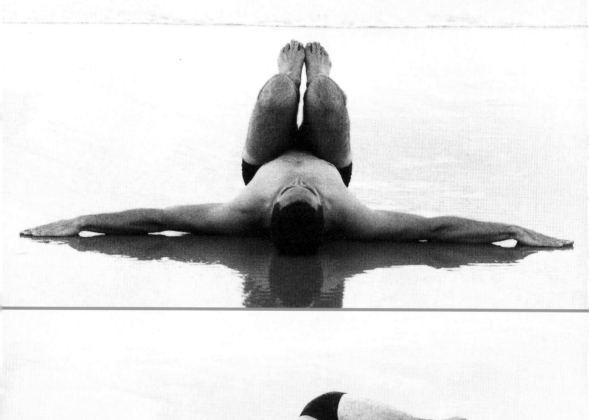
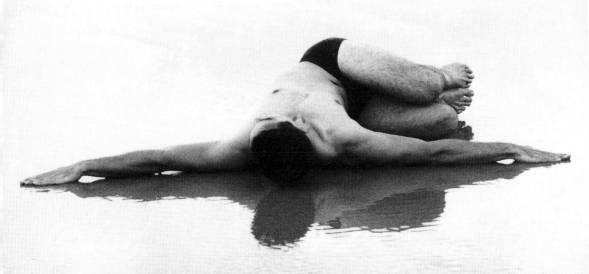

Sukhasana Twist

SUKHA — HAPPY

Positioning: Sit cross-legged. Place your right hand on the ground behind your right hip. Place your left arm on your right knee. Inhale and lift out of your waist. Exhale and turn to look over your right shoulder.

Breathing: As you inhale, lift out of your hips, thinning your waist. As you exhale, turn deeper into the spinal twist.

Focus: Keep your eye gaze over your right shoulder to the far right.

Hold: For five breaths. Release and repeat the posture on the other side.

Benefits: This posture tones the spinal cord, stretches the spinal muscles and separates the vertebrae. It also stimulates blood circulation through the spine and opens the hips.

For an instant pep-up this refreshing twist can be performed any time of the day to release tension in the neck, shoulders and back.

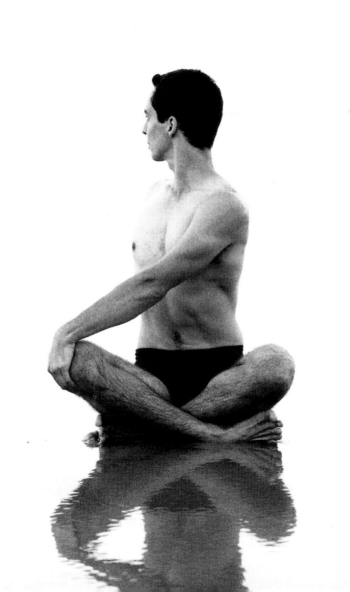

Backbends rejuvenate the body and mind. As they open the chest and heart they release negative emotions and stimulate a positive state of mind.

Having a strong, supple back is integral to good health. The nervous system travels through the spine to every organ. Backbends open and lengthen the spine, helping to prevent it from degenerating and shortening. The spinal cord is stimulated and oxygenated blood is circulated to all the organs. Stretching the stomach muscles cleanses and tones the internal abdominal organs. The brain receives oxygenated blood which energises a sluggish mind.

Counterbalance backbends with a simple forward bend such as Child Pose to soften and release back muscles and calm the nervous system.

Prevent dizziness caused by moving in and out of the backbends by resting between postures.

It's not advisable to practise backward-bending postures if you have a weak heart, high blood pressure or if you are pregnant or menstruating.

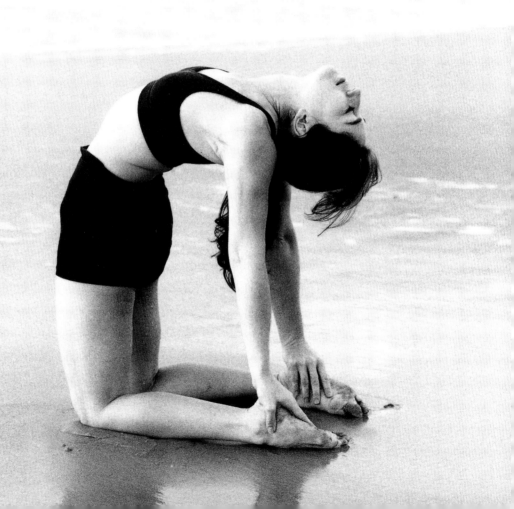

Urdhva Mukha Svanasana

URDHVA – UPWARD; MUKHA – FACE; SVANA – DOG

Positioning: Lie on your stomach with your legs straight and your elbows bent to place your hands beside your shoulders. Rest your forehead on the floor. Inhale and raise your head, shoulders and chest off the ground. Squeeze your buttocks and extend out of your lower back. Straighten your arms and roll your shoulders back and down. Open your chest. Drop your head back and start to work into the backbend with your breath. Lift out of your lower back. Look up to your third eye (the point between your eyebrows).

Breathing: As you exhale, gently release deeper into the backbend. Breathe deeply and slowly.

Focus: Send your eye gaze up to your third eye, stretching the front of your body and focusing inward.

Hold: For five breaths.

Benefits: This posture keeps the back supple and healthy, regenerates the muscles of the torso and relieves back pain, helping slipped discs. It also massages the abdominal organs and stimulates and tones the sexual organs.

This backward-bending *asana* relieves backache and develops a supple spine. The chest opens out, encouraging deep, full breathing.

92

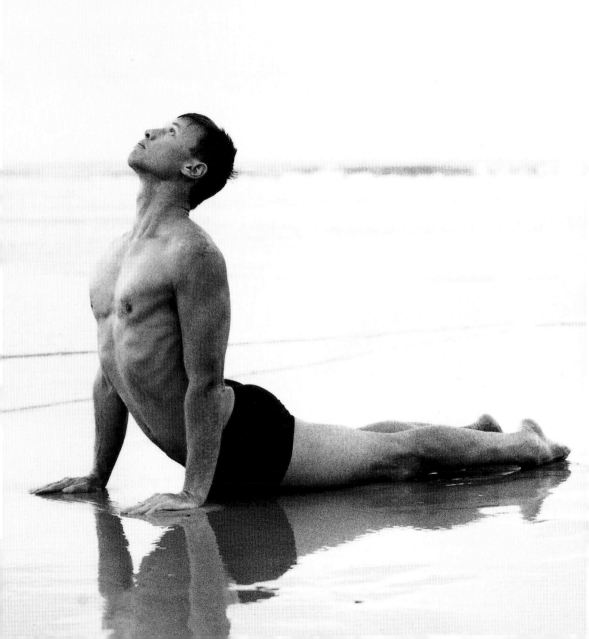

Salabhasana

SALABHA — LOCUST

Positioning: Lie on your stomach with your legs straight and your arms resting alongside your body. Place the backs of your hands on the floor. Rest your forehead on the floor. Inhale fully and raise your head, chest, arms and legs off the floor. Breathe normally as you hold the position and raise a little higher. Squeeze your buttocks and keep your legs together and straight as you lift.

Breathing: Inhale to raise up; exhale to release down. Breathe normally as you hold the position.

Focus: Keep your legs together and open your chest.

Hold: For five breaths.

Variations: Try raising just your head, chest and arms off the floor or just your legs, with your arms, chest and head resting. Alternatively, raise one arm only, then change sides, or raise one leg only and then change sides.

Benefits: This posture strengthens the chest and heart, massages and cleanses the kidneys, liver, intestines and other abdominal organs and stimulates the intestines for healthy bowel function. It aids in eliminating diseases of the stomach, strengthens the spine and tones the nerves of the spine and limbs.

Precautions: Do not practise this posture if you have a weak heart or a hernia.

The body lifts to form a small arch. All the muscles at the back of the body lift and strengthen, helping develop a strong, healthy back.

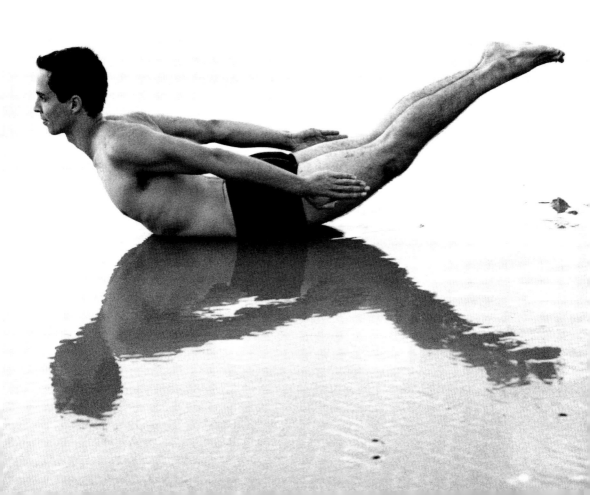

Mini Backbend

Positioning: Lie on your back. Bend your legs. Place your feet up to your buttocks, hip width apart. Extend your arms alongside your body with the palms facing down. Exhale and slowly roll up off the floor. Get in touch with each vertebra as you roll up. First lift your buttocks, then your lower back, middle back and chest. Keep your shoulders down. Squeeze your buttocks and lift your hips up high.

Breathing: Exhale to come into and out of the full posture. Breathe normally as you hold the pose.

Focus: Send your eye gaze down to your navel, opening your chest, lifting your hips and keeping your knees in toward each other.

Hold: For five breaths.

Benefits: This posture massages the abdominal muscles and organs and stimulates blood flow through the spine. It keeps the spine supple, elastic and revitalised, the pelvic organs healthy, and tones the legs and buttocks.

This backward bend helps the spine and the whole body to regenerate rather than degenerate, keeping it stretched, supple and full of life.

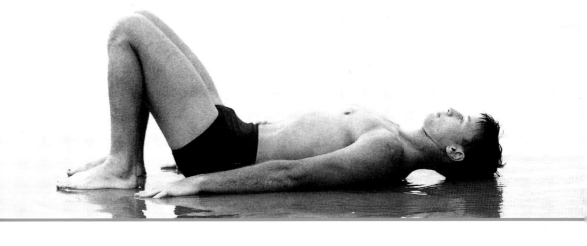

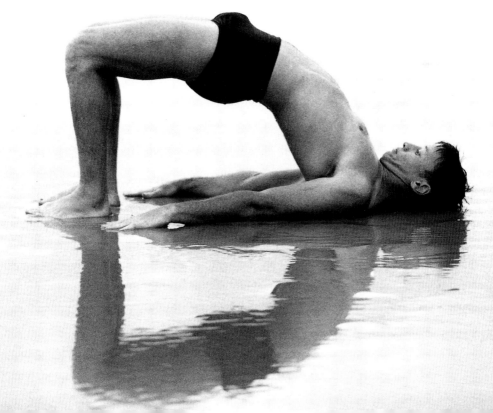

Inverted postures stimulate the flow of pure oxygenated blood to the whole body. Blockages in the organs, muscles and nerves are cleared and the body works more effectively. The oxygen supply increases and the body receives more 'life force'.

Stress and anxiety are reduced as the increased circulation flushes out toxins and purifies the glands, improving the functioning of the body. Accumulated wastes in the legs are removed and replenished with fresh, energising blood. The breathing slows down and deepens, and the intake of oxygen increases with the outflow of carbon dioxide.

The inverted postures are great stimulants for the brain. Being upside down, more pure oxygenated blood is directed to the brain. Consequently, the mind is invigorated and refreshed.

It is not advisable to practise inverted postures if you have high blood pressure or a weak heart. Do not practise *Salamba Sarvangasana* if you are menstruating or pregnant.

Inverted postures

Adho Mukha Svanasana

ADHO – DOWNWARD; MUKHA – FACE; SVANA – DOG

Positioning: Kneel on the ground. Place your hands on the ground in front of your knees and spread your fingers wide apart. Step your right foot back, then your left foot. Straighten your legs, with your feet hip width apart. Inhale and raise your buttocks and hips. Lower the crown of your head toward the floor. Relax your neck and lift your shoulders back and toward your ears. Release your chest through your shoulders, and work your heels to the ground.

Breathing: Breathe deeply in the posture.

Focus: Keep your eyes focused between your feet on the floor, opening your shoulders, and lifting your hips and buttocks. Focus also on locking your knees, opening the backs of your legs and keeping the palm and heel of your hands pressed to the floor with your fingers spread evenly apart.

Hold: For five to ten breaths. Exhale to release out of the posture.

Variations: Place your head on a bolster for a resting pose and keep your knees bent if your legs are tight.

Benefits: This posture strengthens the arms, tones the sciatic nerve and stretches the ankles and backs of the legs.

Precaution: It is not advisable to practise this posture is you have high blood pressure.

Each limb is stretched out in this posture. The inverted position calms the mind and nervous system and cleanses and massages the internal organs.

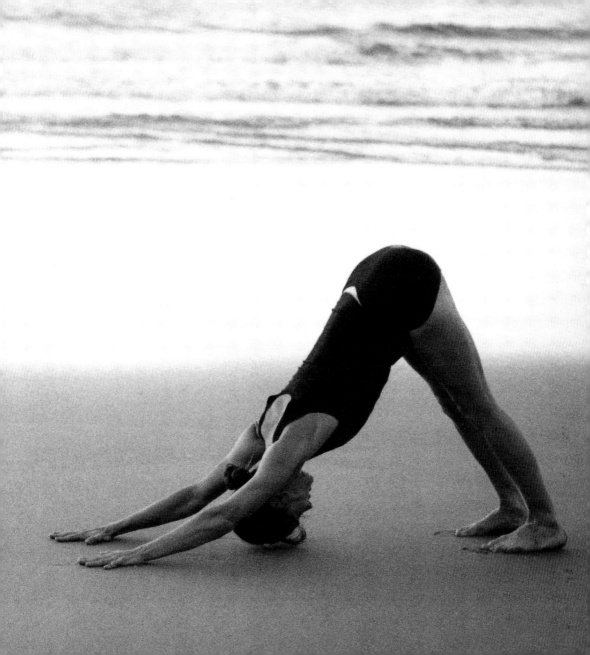

Inverted Legs I, II and III

Positioning: Lie flat on your back with your legs up against the wall. Press the buttocks firmly into the wall. Press your lower back to the floor. Gently activate your leg muscles. Rest the back of your hands on the floor and tuck in your chin.

Breathing: Breathe through your nose softly and slowly. This will calm your whole body.

Focus: Close your eyes (or cover your eyes with an eye pad for deep relaxation) and feel the blood flowing down through your legs.

Hold: For five minutes or as long as it feels good. To release out of the posture, bring your knees to your chest and roll to the side.

Benefits: This posture relieves tired feet and legs and refreshes the mind.

Variations: In Inverted Legs II, spread your legs apart. This stimulates blood flow to the hips, pelvis and reproductive organs, and stretches the inner leg muscles. For Inverted Legs III, bend your knees and place the soles of your feet together. The hips open and blood flows to the reproductive organs.

Fatigue and sluggishness are washed away by pure, oxygenated blood and replaced with vitality and alertness.

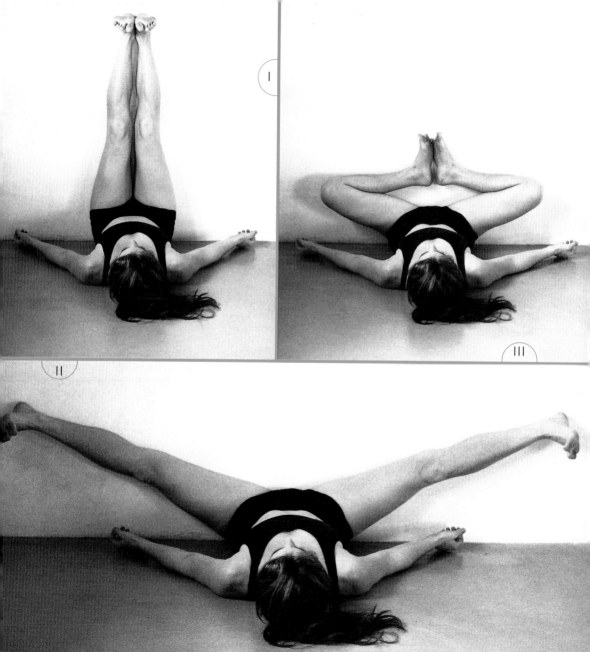

Salamba Sarvangasana

SALAMBA — SUPPORTED; SARVANGASANA — BODY BALANCE

Positioning: Make a neat pile of two or three blankets and lie with your back and shoulders on it. Rest your head onto the floor. Bend your knees and bring your feet into your buttocks. Raise your legs off the floor and place the palms of your hands into your upper back for lift and support. Bring your legs into a vertical position, forming a straight line with your legs and torso. The elbows should sit at shoulder width apart, and the elbows, upper arms and shoulders together support the body. Tuck in your chin and keep your legs lifting.

Breathing: Use normal breathing.

Focus: Keep your eye gaze on your navel. Concentrate on the sound of your breathing, relaxing your head and neck and keeping your body steady and straight.

Hold: For a few breaths. If pressure develops in the head or eyes, come out of the pose immediately. Exhale to release down, remove the blankets and rest with your body flat on the floor. Do not turn your head or neck in this posture.

Salamba Sarvangasana continued over the page

This shoulder stand is known as the 'mother *asana*' for its powerful healing and calming effects on the systems of the entire body.

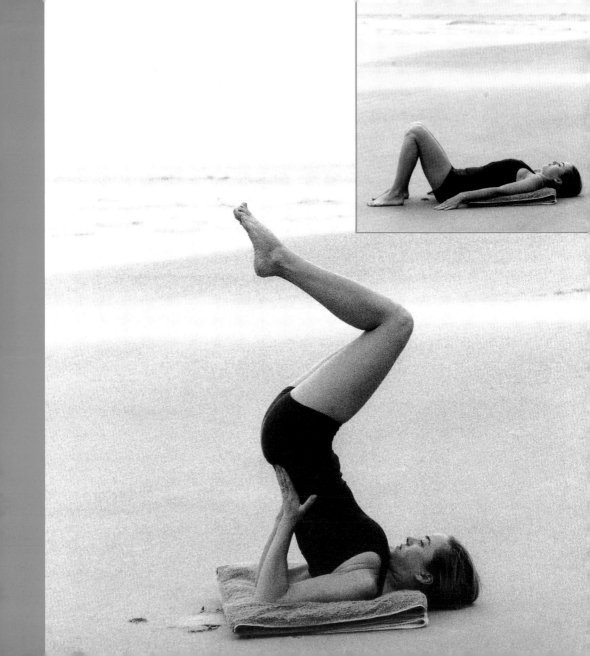

Benefits: This posture relieves mental and physical fatigue and improves the functioning of the circulatory, digestive, nervous, glandular and reproductive systems. It supplies the brain with plenty of oxygenated blood, stimulates the thyroid gland and tones the muscles of the arms, legs and spine. It also stimulates the elimination of fats around the waist, massages the abdominal and reproductive organs and promotes healthy bowel function.

Precautions: It is not advisable to practise this posture if you have a weak heart, high blood pressure or if you are pregnant or menstruating. Ask for assistance from a qualified yoga teacher before attempting this posture for the first time on your own.

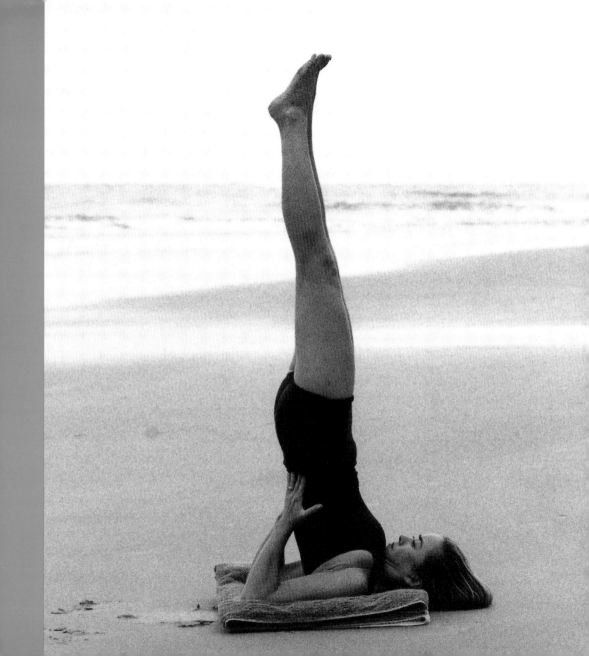

Relaxation postures are a restful 'retreat' for the body, mind and soul. They will leave you feeling completely rejuvenated.

All body systems rest. The nerves relax completely, and muscles release stored tension.

The sound of the breath is the main focal point. The mind learns to empty itself of busy thoughts and develop concentration.

By practising conscious relaxation, the mind and body ultimately perform better in everyday life. Our interaction with the world improves, along with our feelings of inner peace.

For sufferers of anxiety and stress who find being relaxed, still and quiet truly difficult, the following relaxation *asanas* will help give the body and mind the rest they need so much.

Practise the relaxation postures in a warm and quiet environment away from any distractions. The use of an eye pad to cover your eyes deepens relaxation, relieving tired eye muscles.

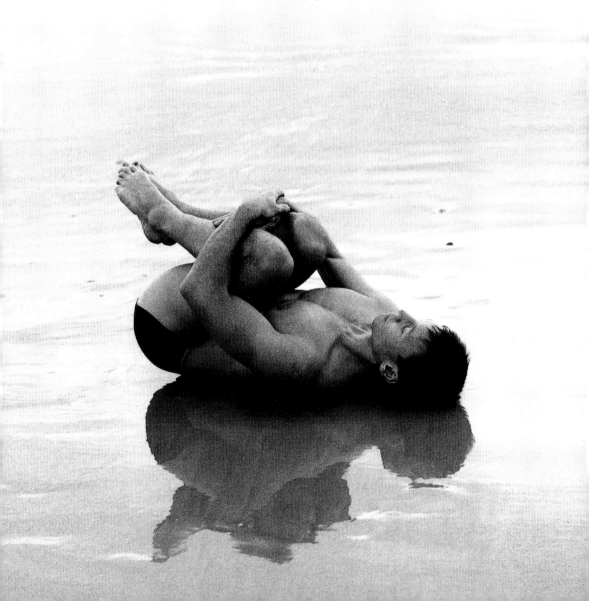

Savasana I

SAVA — LIFELESS BODY

Positioning: Lie flat on your back with your arms slightly away from your body and your palms facing upward. Have your legs separated a little and let the feet fall toward the floor. Tuck in your chin slightly. Adjust your body so that it feels centred and comfortable and close your eyes. Bring your awareness to any part of your body that is tense and relax that area. Resolve not to move your body throughout the practice. Feel your body sinking through the floor, deeper and deeper into relaxation, but do not allow yourself to fall asleep.

Breathing: Slow and rhythmic.

Focus: Observe your breath. Whenever you find yourself thinking, return your awareness to your breath. Relax the muscles of your whole body, from the muscles of your scalp, your face, and down to your toes.

Hold: For ten minutes at the end of every yoga practice, or for a few minutes between postures, especially after dynamic postures. To release from the pose, roll to the right, then slowly come up to a sitting position.

Variations: Cover your eyes with an eye bag to relax your eye muscles and relieve headache. You can also use a small pillow to rest your head on or to place under your knees if lying flat is uncomfortable for your back.

Benefits: This posture relaxes the entire body, rests the nervous system and quietens the mind. It develops concentration and awareness and aids in relieving insomnia if practised before sleeping.

The body is completely still; there is no movement apart from the breathing. The mind is awake to the delicious experience of deep relaxation.

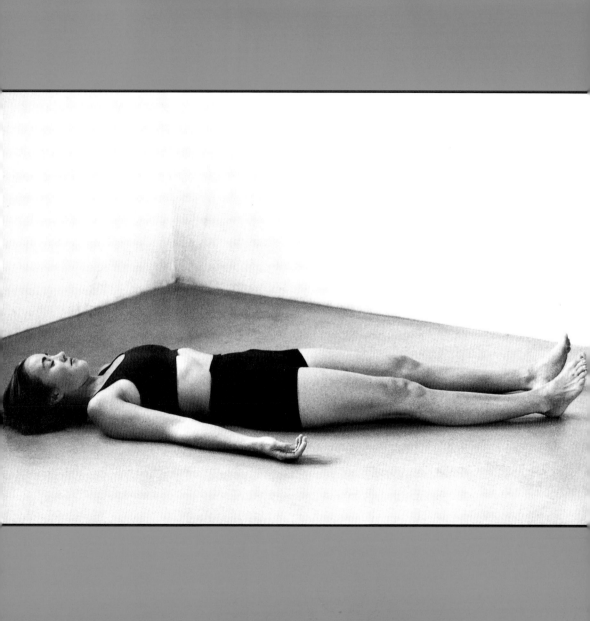

Savasana II

SAVA — LIFELESS BODY

Positioning: Use a bolster or place two or three blankets into a neat pile and fold one blanket in half for a head rest. Sit on the floor with your buttocks touching the edge of the bolster. Stretch your legs out and lower your body down over the bolster, opening your chest. Rest your head on the folded blanket and tuck in your chin. The buttocks stay on the floor and the chest opens. With your body now completely relaxed, listen to your breath. Feel your chest rising as you inhale and sinking as you exhale.

Breathing: Take deep, slow, full breaths through your nose.

Focus: The eyes are closed. Focus on your third eye (the point between your eyebrows). This point of focus develops awareness and intuition. Listen to the sound of your breath and relax every muscle in your body.

Hold: For five to ten minutes. To release slowly, roll to rest on your right side, then come up to a sitting position.

Benefits: This posture relaxes the entire body, rests the nervous system and quietens the mind. It purifies the heart and lungs, improves respiratory functions and develops concentration and awareness. Practised before sleeping, this posture helps eliminate insomnia.

This supported relaxation posture opens the chest, enabling deeper breathing and deep relaxation.

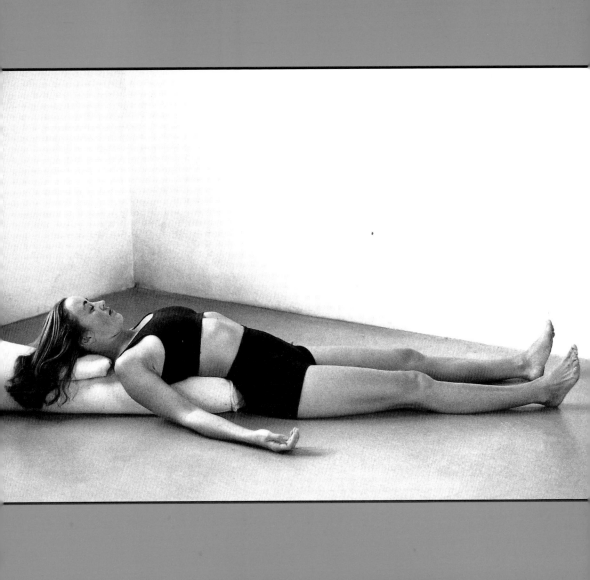

Savasana III

SAVA – LIFELESS BODY

Positioning: Lie on your stomach and rest your forehead on the floor or turn your head to one side. Stretch your arms forward above your head and relax the muscles of your whole body.

Breathing: Breathe slowly through the nose.

Focus: Have your eyes closed and focus on the sound of your breath.

Hold: For ten minutes at the end of a session of *asanas* or for a few minutes in between yoga postures. To release, roll to rest on your right side, then slowly come up to a sitting position.

Benefits: *Savasana III* improves posture, extends the spine and helps to prevent slipped discs. It relieves tension in the spinal muscles and relaxes the mind.

This resting posture is good for sleeping. The stomach is gently soothed, the arms extend above the head and the spine gently stretches.

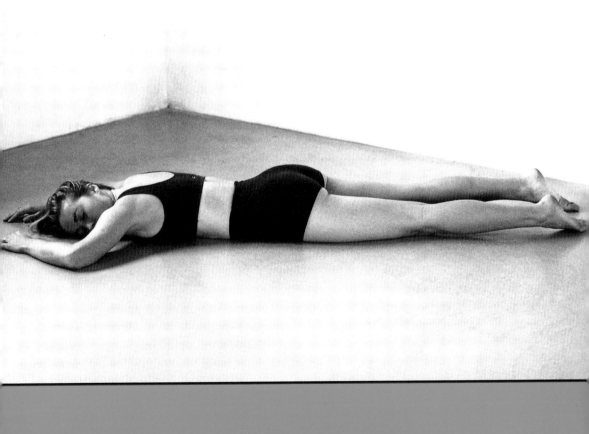

Supta Baddha Konasana

SUPTA – SUPINE; BADDHA – BOUND; KONA – ANGLE

Positioning: Place a bolster or two folded blankets horizontally. Sit on the floor with your lower back touching the bolster, bend your knees and bring the soles of your feet together. Lie back over the bolster, rest your head on the floor and tuck in your chin. Your knees will drop down and your hips will open. Rest the bent arms on the floor alongside your head. Feel your abdomen extending over the bolster. Close your eyes.

Breathing: Breathe slowly and evenly through your nose.

Focus: On the sound of your breath.

Hold: For five minutes. Inhale to release up out of the posture.

Variations: Place your arms down alongside your body, with your palms facing upward. If your back is stiff, lie over the bolster lengthways, supporting your head and neck. For a more intense opening in your hips, use a belt. From the sitting position place the middle of the belt around your sacrum and the two ends over your thighs, knees and shins. Tie the belt under your feet. Keep the belt low on your back, firmly but not too tightly, and lie back over the bolster.

Benefits: This posture relaxes the whole body, opens the chest and encourages healthy breathing. It loosens the hip muscles, massages the abdominal organs, stimulates blood to the reproductive and sexual organs, promotes a healthy menstrual cycle and relieves menstrual pain.

This deeply relaxing posture opens the chest and massages the internal organs. The hips lie open, increasing the supply of blood to the pelvic and reproductive organs.

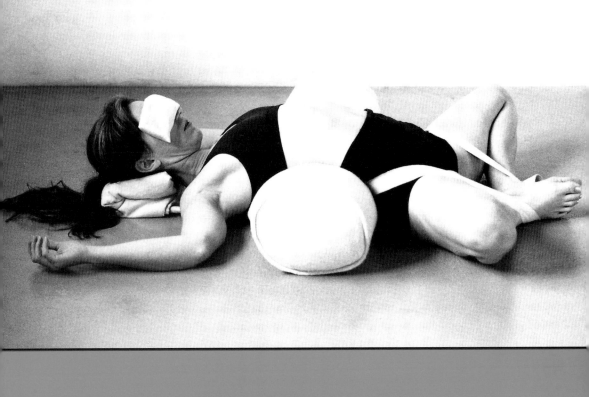

Child Pose

Positioning: Sit with your buttocks on your heels. Rest your torso on your knees, and the backs of your arms alongside your legs with the palms facing upward. Rest your forehead on the floor, drop your shoulders and relax every muscle in your body. Feel your head and body sinking into deep relaxation.

Breathing: Breathe slowly and naturally.

Focus: Keep your eyes closed and rest your body.

Hold: For a few minutes between postures when the body needs resting. Inhale to release.

Variation: Rest your head on a bolster.

Benefits: This posture calms the mind, and slows the breath and heart rate, cooling the body.

Symbolic of a curled-up child, warm and protected from the outside world, this posture offers a nurturing and restful space.

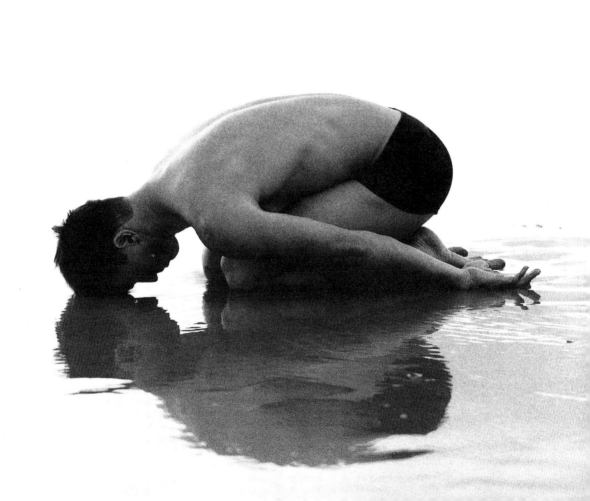

Knee Hug

Positioning: Lie on your back. Hug your knees to your chest, while you keep your head, neck and shoulders relaxed and on the floor.

Breathing: Use normal breathing.

Focus: Close your eyes or gaze beyond your knees and relax your back muscles.

Hold: For as long as it feels good. Practise this posture after backbends to release the muscles.

Benefits: This posture releases the muscles of the lower back and relaxes the body.

This simple posture softens the back. Hug the knees into the chest to release and relax tight, spasming lower back muscles.

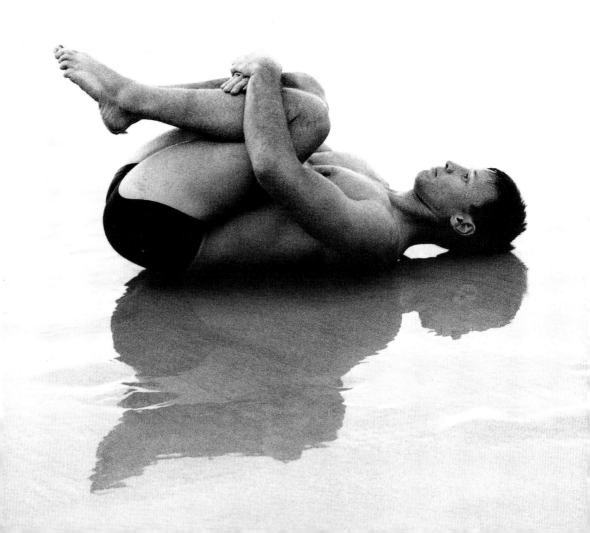

Forward Rest

Positioning: Kneel on the floor. Bring your big toes together with the knees apart. Sit your buttocks back between your heels, onto the soles of your feet. Cup your fingers onto the floor in front, and inhale and lengthen out of your hips. Exhale and slowly release forward and down, walking your arms forward as you are extending and rest your forehead onto the floor. Keep your buttocks back to your heels and stretch your arms forward, spreading your fingers. Feel the two-way stretch of your spine: your shoulders and arms are stretching your upper back forward and your buttocks are working the lower back backward.

Breathing: Breathe deep, slow, full breaths through the nose.

Focus: Close your eyes, and focus your third eye (the point between your eyebrows), resting your body and mind and keeping your buttocks back toward your heels.

Hold: For as long as it is comfortable, and for a few minutes after a backbend to release tight muscles.

Variation: Turn your head to the side if your neck feels sore.

Benefits: This posture separates the vertebrae of the spine, promoting a supple healthy back. It also cools the body and relaxes the mind.

This is a gentle forward-resting *asana* that stretches, lengthens and straightens the spine. The forehead sinks to the floor, calming the activity of the mind.

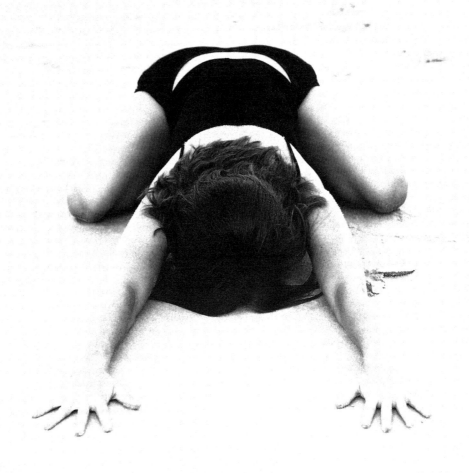

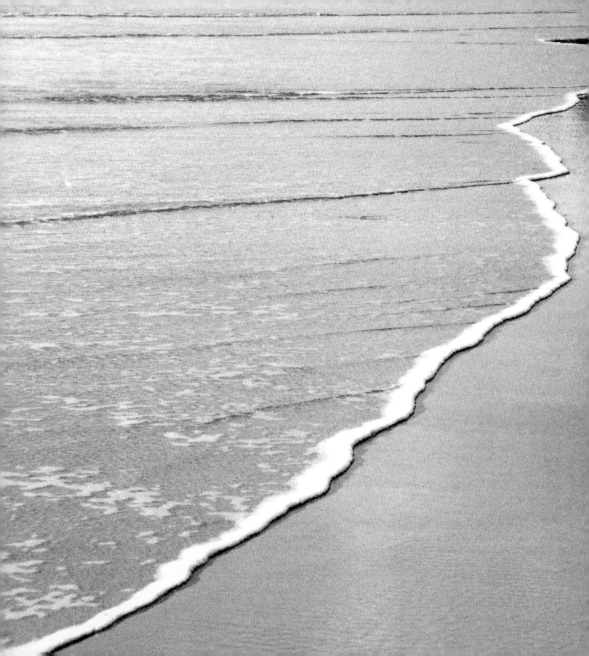

Deep Relaxation

The following method of relaxation is designed to relax your body and mind, and release stress. It is a delicious technique that calms the mind and rejuvenates the soul. This kind of relaxation is a great way to wind down and return to your centre after a busy day at work.

The process involves isolating each part of the body and consciously relaxing it. We move through the whole body, becoming more aware of tense areas. We release tension and hold in the muscles until the whole body is completely soft and relaxed.

Positioning: Choose a quiet environment away from any distractions. Take the phone off the hook and ask others not to disturb you.

Lie in *Savasana I* (page 110) and make sure you are warm and comfortable. You may like to use a pillow, blankets and eye bag for more comfort.

Become aware of your whole body lying on the floor. Starting on the right side, become aware of your right thumb. Relax it completely. Feel any tensions moving out of the thumb.

Now take your awareness to the second finger and relax it. Relax the third finger, fourth finger, then little finger. Relax all your fingers. Relax the palm of your hand, then the back of your hand. Feel your whole hand relaxed and soft, sinking into the floor.

Take your awareness to your wrist and release the muscles and joints in it. Then release your right forearm, elbow, upper arm and armpit. Relax your whole right arm completely.

Now move your awareness to your right foot. Relax your big toe, second toe, third toe, fourth toe and little toe. Relax the top of your foot, the ball and heel of your foot, then the inner arch. Relax your whole foot.

Relax your ankle, and then your lower leg. Relax the front of your knee, the back of your knee, the thigh, the back of your leg. Relax your whole right leg. Feel that the whole leg is soft and completely relaxed.

Now take your awareness to the right side of your torso. Relax your right hip, buttock, then the right side of your waist. Relax your chest, then your right shoulder.

Relax your whole torso. Relax your whole right side: arm, leg, torso.

Now repeat on your left side, starting with your hand, then leg and torso.

Then move your attention to your head and relax your whole head, neck and face into the floor.

Relax your scalp and every muscle in your face. Feel your skin falling away from the bone and your head sinking to the floor. Relax your eyes, nose, mouth; have your lips slightly parted. Relax your tongue, throat and jaw; then your cheek bones and your ears.

Feel that your head and your whole body is completely relaxed.

With your entire body relaxed, feel yourself sinking deeper and deeper into a state of complete relaxation. Ahhh ...

Breathing: Use normal, soft breathing through your nose.

Focus: Feel every muscle in the body relaxing, releasing tension in the muscles, and the whole body sinking. Whenever you find yourself thinking, return to the point of focus.

Hold: For as long as it is comfortable. Five to ten minutes is effective.

Benefits: This posture is extremely healing for stressed-out anxious minds. It calms the whole nervous system and relaxes the body and mind.

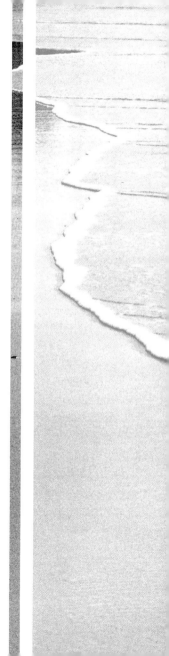

Meditation is yoga in its highest form. It is the experience of emptiness, a holiday for the mind.

Regular meditation, whether for five minutes or an hour, makes you more cheerful and positive. Your mind becomes clear and focused.

Meditation is about being totally in the moment. In practising yoga, become aware of every breath and body movement. This itself is meditation.

The senses are withdrawn from the world and the mind focuses inward. Begin by focusing on the soft sound of your breath or reciting a mantra (a prayerful word or phrase). Then let all your thoughts and worries go. Give yourself the ultimate gift, time to relax.

Meditation can be practised any time. The very early morning is ideal. It is also often easier after activities like dancing, walking or yoga when the body is relaxed and the mind has already been concentrating inwardly on the body and breath.

Meditation postures

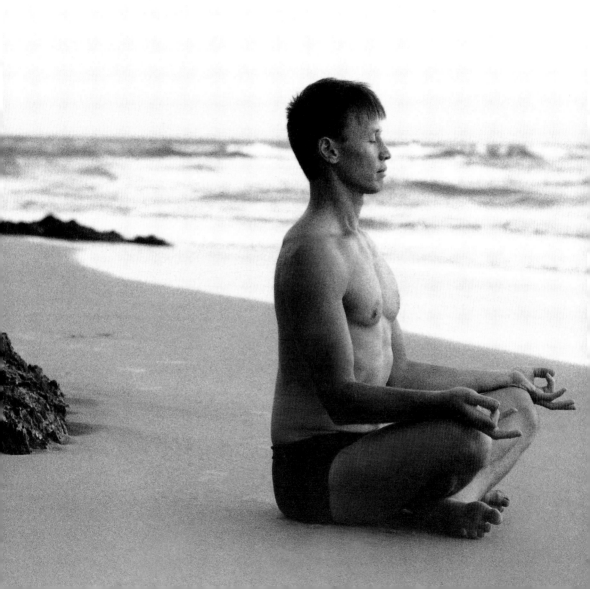

Sukhasana Meditation

SUKHA — HAPPY

Positioning: Bend the forefinger of each hand and place it behind the nail of the thumb. Relax your other three fingers so they spread apart. (This hand posture is called *Jnana Mudra*. The nerve impulses of the forefinger turn inward and help to relax the body.) Sit on a neat pile of blankets and lightly cross the legs. Roll the shoulders down and back to open out the chest. Rest the backs of the hands on the tops of the knees.

Breathing: Use normal breathing.

Focus: Close your eyes. Find a point of focus you are comfortable with, such as the soft sound of your breath or the sensation of cool air moving in through your nostrils and warm air moving out. Whenever you lose focus, return your awareness to the focal point. Keep your head and back straight.

Hold: The longer the better. After a session of yoga, practise meditation for a few minutes before lying down into a version of *Savasana*.

Variations: Sit with your back against a wall for support if your back muscles are weak. Tie a cloth around your eyes to help draw your attention inward. Wrap a cloth firmly around your abdomen and lower back to draw the spine erect.

Benefits: Relaxing and meditating is known to promote clarity of thought and give you a more positive outlook on life. It helps you feel more rejuvenated and alive.

130

This is an easy position to sit in for meditation. The body is comfortable and the spine and head are aligned. Drawing the awareness inward comes effortlessly.

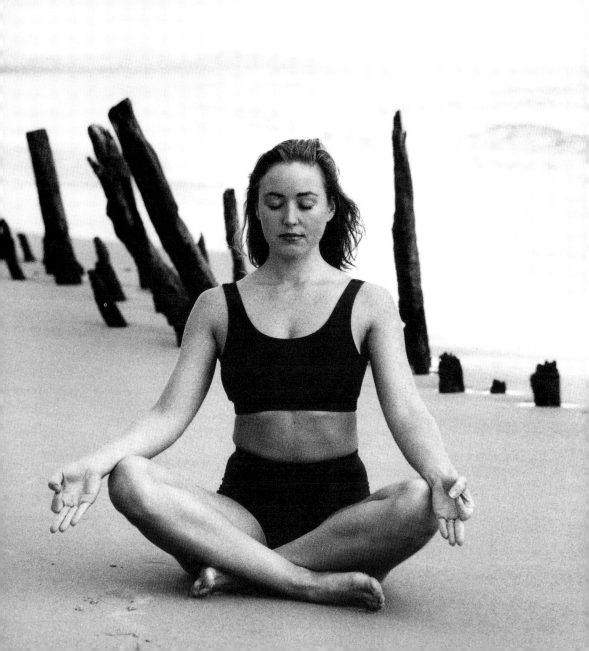

Half Lotus

Positioning: Sit in *Sukhasana*. Cross the left leg over the right. Raise the right foot out and place it on top of the left upper thigh. The right leg is now on top. The right knee sits over the left foot. Feel the hips opening. Sit the buttocks onto a neat pile of blankets if that is more comfortable. Rest the backs of your hands on your knees and bend your forefingers to rest behind the nails at the thumb. The other fingers relax completely. Close your eyes and bring your awareness to a quiet space within.

Breathing: Use normal breathing.

Hold: The longer the better. After a session of yoga, practise meditation for a few minutes before lying down into a version of *Savasana*.

Focus: Close your eyes and free your mind of thoughts. Focus on keeping your back upright.

Benefits: Sitting with the back straight promotes healthy posture and circulation. Time stands still as your focus is drawn inward.

When your thoughts wander, let them go and return your focus to the soft sound of your breath.

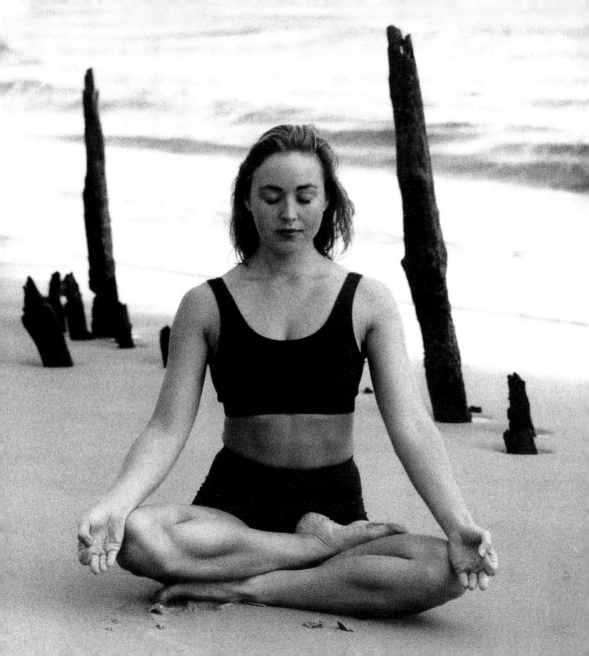

Virasana Meditation

VIRA — A HERO

Positioning: Sit with the knees bent and the buttocks resting back onto the heels. Keep the knees and feet together. Rest the backs of the hands on the knees. Bend the forefingers and rest the nails behind the thumb. Let the other fingers relax outward. Close the eyes and draw your awareness within.

Breathing: Use normal breathing.

Hold: For as long as you like. Practise meditation after a session of yoga before lying back into a version of *Savasana*.

Focus: Close your eyes. Find a point of focus you are comfortable with, such as the soft sound of your breath or the sensation of cool air moving in through your nostrils and warm air moving out. Whenever you find your thoughts wandering, return your awareness to the focal point. Keep your head and back straight.

Benefits: This deeply relaxing posture promotes clear thinking and rejuvenates the mind. You will feel alive and refreshed afterwards.

Variations: Lean up against a wall if your back becomes tired. Keep lifting your torso upward.

When the body is still and the mind is free of thought, then there is an empty space to be at peace.

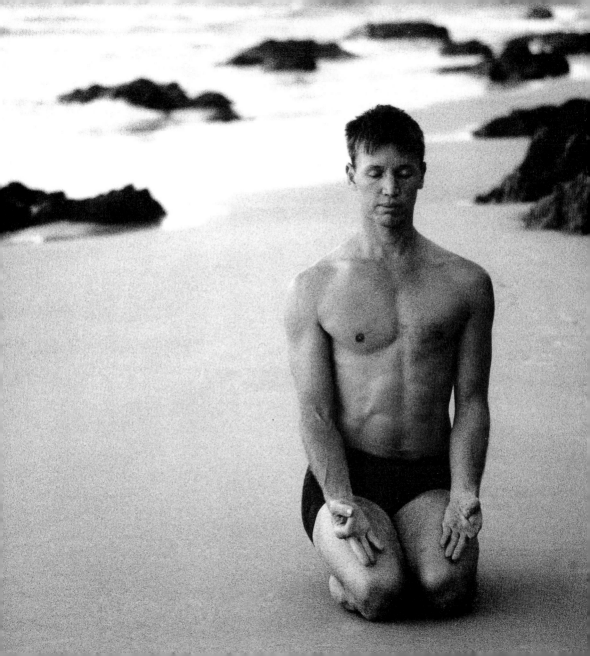

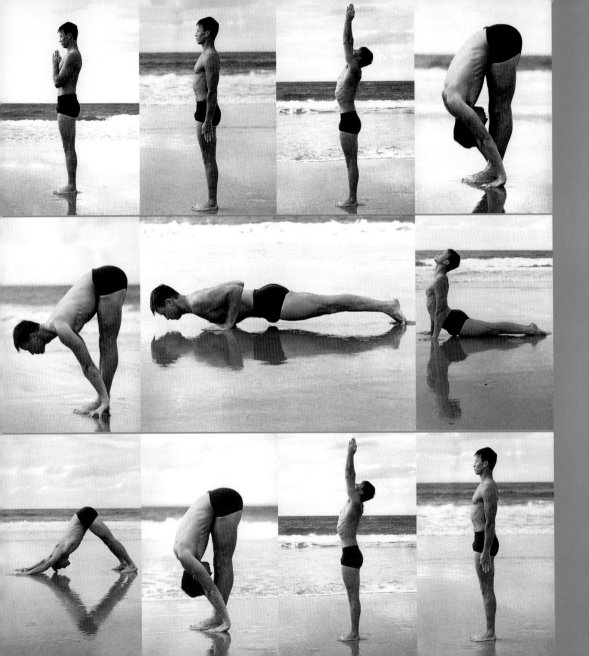

Simple sequences

Greeting the day, or *Surya Namaskar*, is an all-over yoga session in one simple sequence. *Surya Namaskar* is traditionally practised at sunrise, a time of inspiration and abundant energy at the start of a new day. This is a dynamic practice in which the body warms up quickly after flowing through a sequence of postures with the breath. The circulation of body heat softens and opens the muscles. Toxins and wastes are released and excess body fat burnt off.

Practise the sequence at any time to refresh your body and mind, or to warm up your body before practising other yoga postures. Keep the rhythm and flow of your breath even, inhaling and exhaling fully into and out of each posture.

With practice, the body will become more flexible and the rhythm of your breathing will improve to help the sequence flow.

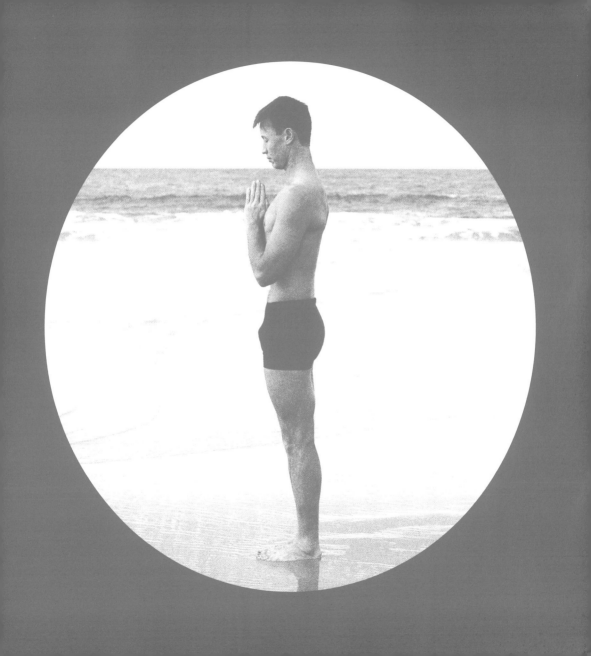

Before beginning the sequence, take time to get in touch with your breathing. Stand with your feet together. Hold your hands in prayer position in front of your heart and relax your whole body. Breathe normally through the nose. Close your eyes and focus on your heart centre. This posture aligns the body and develops concentration.

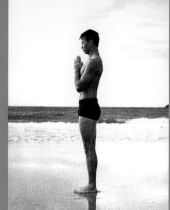

1

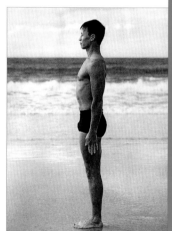

Stand in *Tadasana* (page 28) with your feet together and arms by your side. Look ahead at eye level.

2

Inhale and raise your arms above your head, bringing the palms together. Drop your head back to bring your eye focus up to your hands. The whole body extends upward. Lift your torso from the hips. Focus on the extension of your body. This posture stretches and elongates the body.

3

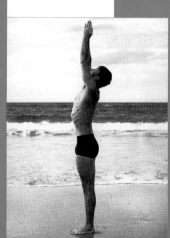

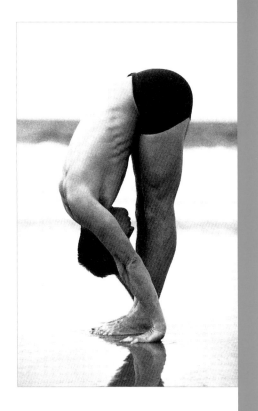

Exhale as you bend at the hips and release your torso down to your legs. As you come down, your arms extend out to the sides. Bring your fingers and hands to the floor, and, if possible, keep your legs straight. If your back is straining, bend your legs slightly. Bring your forehead to your knees. Your eye gaze moves down the body to the point between your navel and pubis. The posture activates the circulation of blood, stretches and tones the spine and spinal cord and stimulates the digestive and excretory systems. It also improves a sluggish stomach, cleanses the liver and kidneys and eliminates fat around the waist.

4

Inhale and look up. Extend your spine so your back straightens, raise your head and look forward. Keep your fingers cupped on the floor beside your feet. Keep your eyes focused ahead, bringing the internal focus to the heart centre, lengthening your spine out of your hips and keeping your legs locked. This posture separates the vertebrae, and tones the spinal cord and nerves of the legs.

5

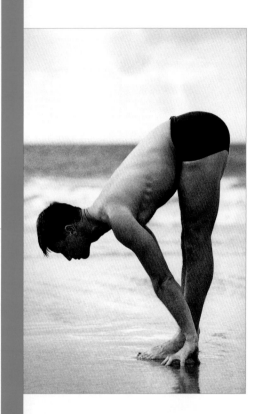

Exhale and step or lightly jump your feet back, releasing down into a plank position. Your arms bend and the elbows stay in close to your body, and your toes are curled under. If you have the strength, keep your body off the floor; if not, rest your body on the floor. Focus your eyes on the tip of your nose and your body in one straight line. This posture strengthens the muscles of the legs and arms.

6

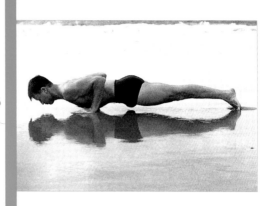

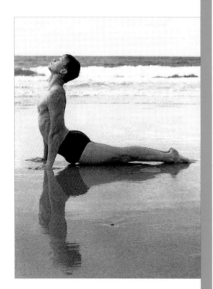

7

As you inhale, roll onto the tops of your feet. Bring the front of your body up through the shoulders, straightening your arms. Drop your head back and arch your back. Keep your legs straight and squeeze your buttocks. Keep your whole body except your hands and feet off the floor, or rest the tops of your legs on the floor. Focus on your third eye, opening your chest, extending from your waist and on lengthening the front of your body. This posture softens and stretches the back, stimulates the spinal nerves and stimulates blood flow to the abdominal organs.

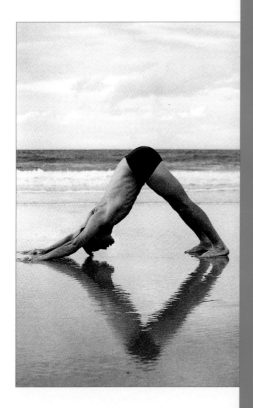

This posture is the resting pose in the sequence. It is held here for five deep, slow breaths. Exhale and lift up your buttocks and hips. Straighten your legs and work your heels back to the floor, with your feet hip width apart. Your hands face forward with the fingers spread wide apart, and your chest and head drop through your shoulders. Keep your eyes focused on a point between your feet on the floor. This posture counterbalances the backbending in the previous posture. The spine stretches and the muscles soften, and the arm and leg muscles stretch and open, stimulating blood flow through the body.

8

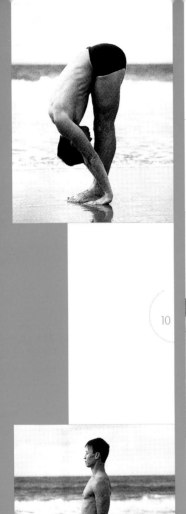

9 Inhale and lightly step or jump your feet to your hands. Look up as in position 5.

Exhale your head down toward your knees. This is the same as position 4.

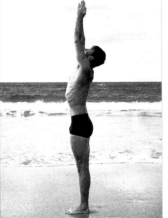

10 Inhale and extend your arms out straight to the sides as you come up to a standing position. Extend your arms up as in position 3.

11 Exhale and release your arms down by the side of your torso. Return your eye focus to a point in front of you as in position 2. Repeat the sequence a few times and try experimenting with the pace.

This half-hour session relieves menstruation pains and restores energy levels whenever you feel exhausted.

For most women, menstruation means low energy levels and changing emotional states. We often have to work when all our body wants is time out and plenty of rest. Listen to what your body is asking for. Take time to restore your energy.

Inverted or strenuous postures are not suitable during menstruation. Practise gentle sitting postures that open the muscles around the hips and pelvis, relieving cramps, heat and tension. The Inverted Leg postures I, II and III on page 102 are safe resting postures since the hips are not raised.

If half an hour is too long, cut out a few postures or reduce the holding time. Always finish a practice with some time in *Savasana*.

Menstruation sequence

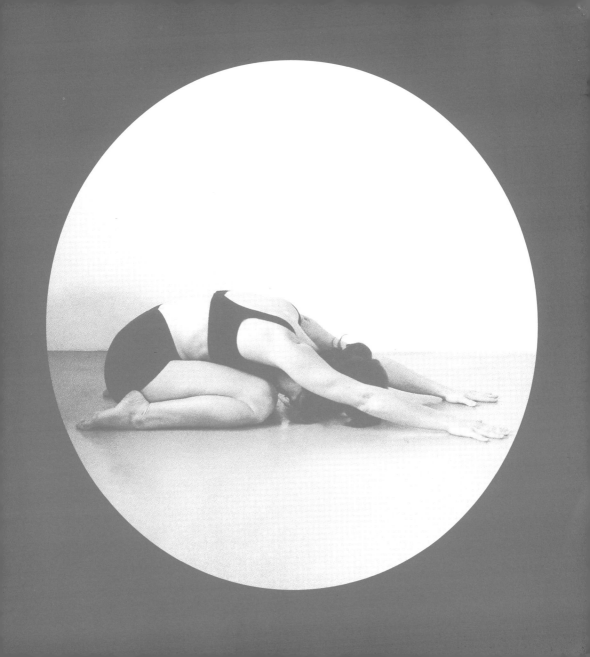

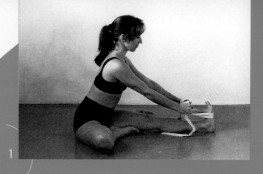

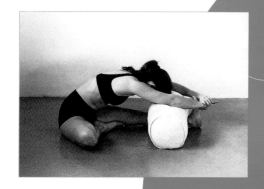

JANU SIRSASANA (page 68)

Practise this posture for one minute on each side. Rest your head on a pillow for variation.

TRIANG MUKHAIKAPADA
PASCIMOTTANASANA (page 70)

Practise this posture for one minute on each side. Rest your head on a pillow for variation.

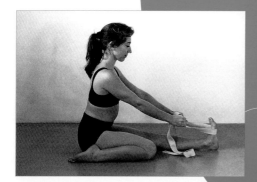

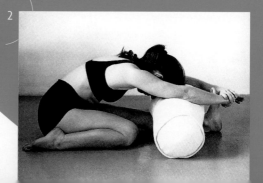

Sit with your legs wide and rest forward with your forehead and arms on a chair for three minutes. This gets the blood circulating, releasing tight hip and pelvic muscles.

3

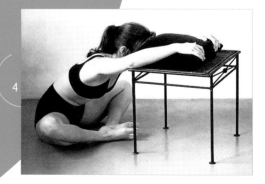

Sit with the soles of your feet together and rest forward with your forehead and arms on a chair for three minutes. Feel the hips softening and the body cooling.

4

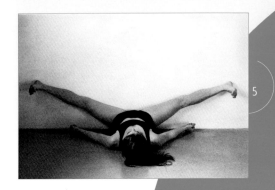

5

INVERTED LEGS II AND III (page 102)
Hold each variation of Inverted Legs for three minutes. These postures are cleansing and rejuvenating. Tired legs and feet are relieved of aches and cramps while the rest of the body relaxes on the floor. The body's systems slow down and help to release stress and anxiety. Feel your energy levels being restored.

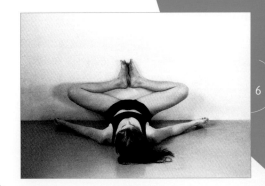

6

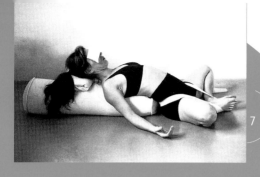

7

SUPTA BADDHA KONASANA (page 116)
Hold this posture for five minutes.

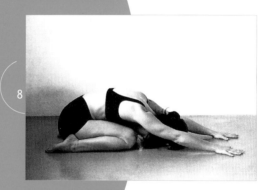

8

VIRASANA II (page 74)
Hold *Virasana I* for three minutes. This posture opens up tight hips and relaxes the body forward and down.

SAVASANA I (page 110)
Lie in *Savasana I* for five to ten minutes. Make sure you are free from distractions. Use an eye bag if you wish to relax more deeply.

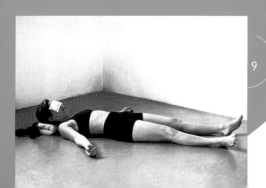

9

This sequence of postures keeps the body and mind healthy and supple during pregnancy and helps you prepare for childbirth. The muscles soften and loosen, keeping the body relaxed and flexible. The back is strengthened and aching legs and feet are relieved of tiredness and cramps.

Get in touch with the breath, breathing deep, full breaths throughout the practice. Make sure your yoga teacher is aware you are pregnant and always advise your medical professional or midwife of the yoga you are practising. Do not practise any postures that cause strain, discomfort or tiredness. Keep the abdomen unconstricted at all times. Do not practise yoga during weeks eleven, twelve or thirteen of your pregnancy and do not exhaust your body in any way.

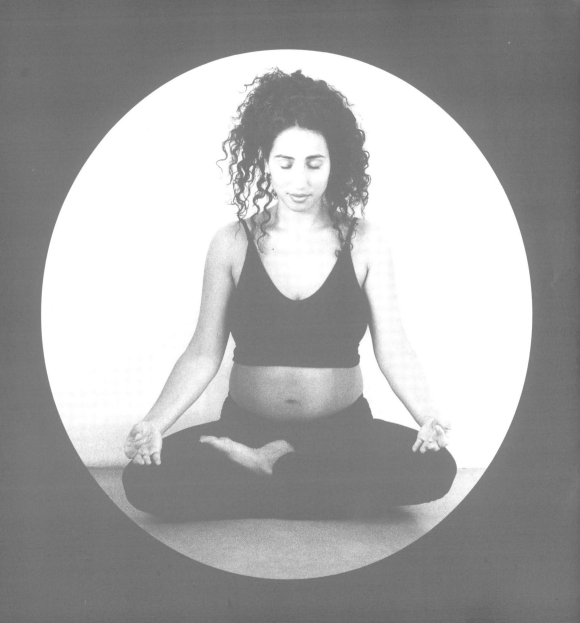

JANU SIRSASANA (page 68)

Use a belt to keep the lower back and abdomen lifting. This strengthens the back muscles which support the increasing weight of the baby. Hold for a minute on each side.

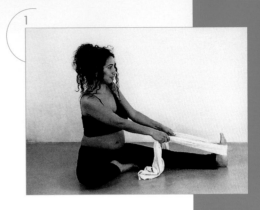

TRIANG MUKHAIKAPADA PASCIMOTTANASANA (page 70)

Keep the back and abdomen lifted and sit the buttock of the outside leg on a blanket for balance. Use a belt or strap. Hold for a minute on each side.

PASCIMOTTANASANA

Sit with the legs outstretched and the back straight. Hold onto a belt and keep the abdomen lifted and unconstricted. Straighten out and stretch the legs. Hold for a few minutes.

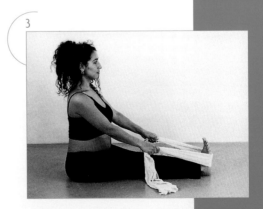

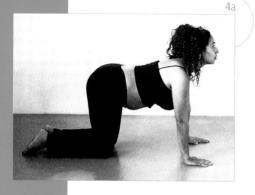

4a

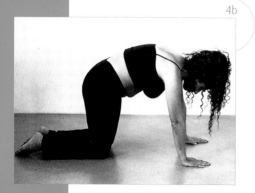

4b

CAT ROLL

This gentle motion of rolling the back down and up gently rocks the baby and relieves lower back pain. First, sit on all fours with the knees hip width apart. Inhale and look up as you lift the buttocks and gently arch the back. (Do not arch the back in the last three months of pregnancy.) With the exhalation, tuck the chin in and under, looking down. Roll the spine up and drop the buttocks. Feel your baby gently rocking and your spine opening and stretching. Move back and forth with the breath. Repeat this motion five times or as much as it is comfortable.

PELVIC SQUAT

Squat down with the feet and knees wide apart. Do not squash the abdomen. Spread the knees wide. Bring the palms together and press the elbows into the knees. The pelvic muscles are activated and strengthened in preparation for the baby's birth. The hips are loosened and stretched. Practise deep, full breathing through the nose. Hold for five to ten breaths.

5

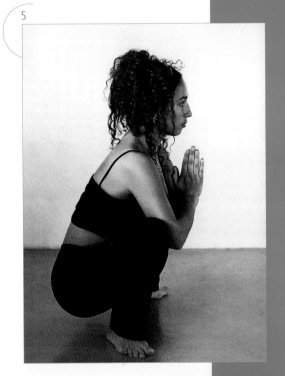

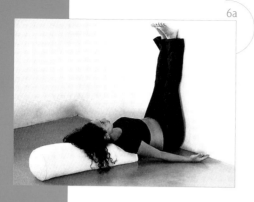

6a

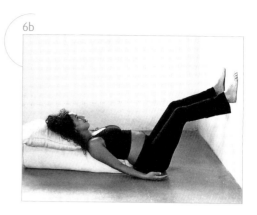

6b

INVERTED LEGS I, II AND III (page 102)

Practise each posture for about three minutes. Use a bolster to support the head, neck, shoulders and back. Practise Inverted Legs II and III if lying with the buttocks against the wall is uncomfortable. In Inverted Legs III, the legs are spread apart. In Inverted Legs III, the knees are bent and the feet rest against the wall. These postures stimulate blood flow to the hips and pelvis and stretch the inner leg muscles.

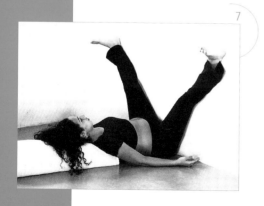

7

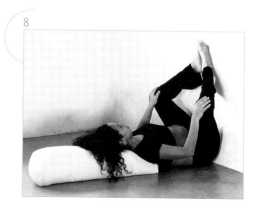

8

SUPTA BADDHA KONASANA (page 116)

Use a bolster or a pillow for this posture. Do not use a belt. Gently place the feet together and let the knees fall open. Relax here for three to five minutes.

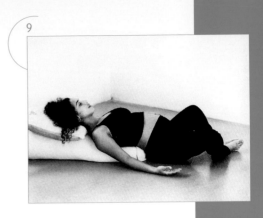

SITTING WITH THE BREATH (page 22)

Lean your back up against a wall for support if it becomes tired. Keep your legs outstretched if sitting cross-legged is uncomfortable. Practise deep, full, relaxed breathing through the nose.

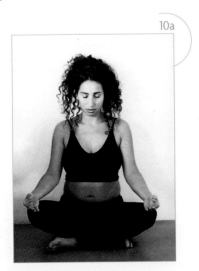

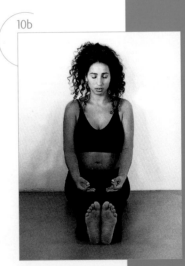

Lie in Savasana II for ten minutes, relaxing the whole body deeply. The chest opens to assist in deep, full breathing. The abdomen opens and is supported. Use a blanket to keep warm and an eye bag if you wish to relax more deeply. Practise this posture in a quiet, warm environment free from distractions.

11

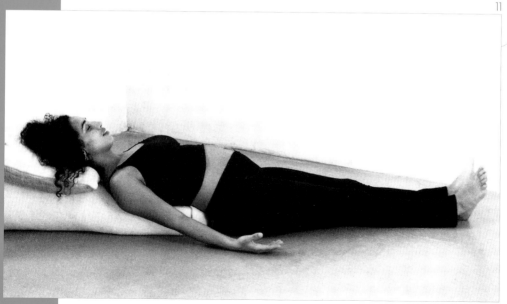

Yoga postures can help you find peace and relief from certain common ailments and conditions. Their therapeutic benefits help to relieve the body and mind of discomfort and anxiety.

The following remedial programs combine particular yoga postures in sequences that will help you with complaints such as backache and tiredness. A qualified yoga teacher will be able to help you further with individual problems. If your condition is serious, seek medical advice before practising.

Try each of the courses so you get to know the sequences that work for you. Always conclude with a version of *Savasana*. If any postures feel wrong or cause strain, slowly release out of the posture. Each courses has twelve postures and takes about twenty-five to thirty minutes.

Remedial courses

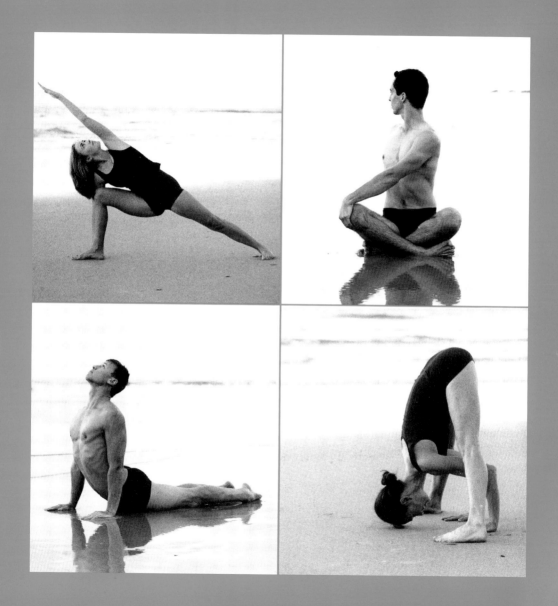

Relieving stress and anxiety

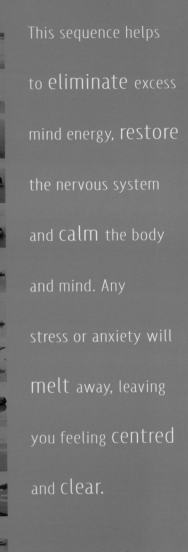

This sequence helps to eliminate excess mind energy, restore the nervous system and calm the body and mind. Any stress or anxiety will melt away, leaving you feeling centred and clear.

162

Practise this sequence when your body is exhausted from a hard day's work. The therapeutic relaxation postures will relieve tiredness and restore your energy levels.

Relieving tiredness

1. *Supta Baddha Konasana*, page 116

2. Inverted Legs I, page 102

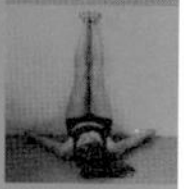

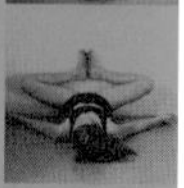

3. Inverted Legs III, page 102

4. Knee Hug, page 120

5. *Uttanasana*, page 48

6. *Virasana II*, page 74

7. *Adho Mukha Svanasana*, page 100

8. *Janu Sirsasana*: head on pillow, page 68

9. *Salamba Sarvangasana*, page 104

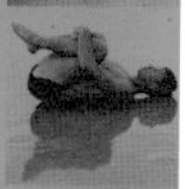

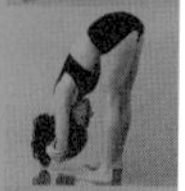

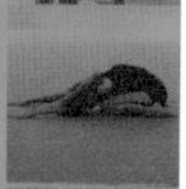

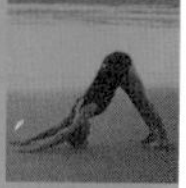

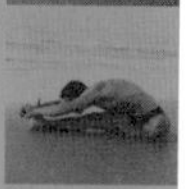

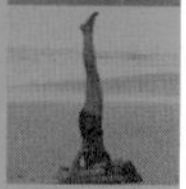

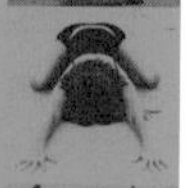

10. Forward Rest, page 122

11. *Sukhasana* Meditation page 130

12. *Savasana II*, page 112

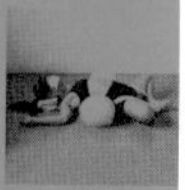

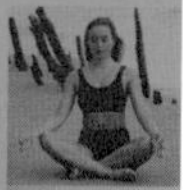

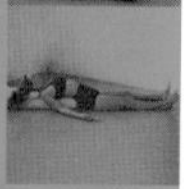

Rejuvenation

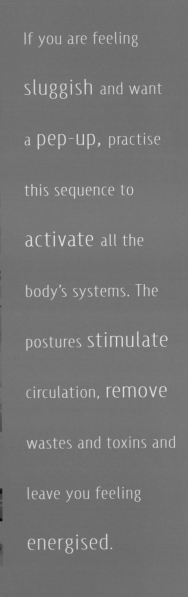

If you are feeling sluggish and want a pep-up, practise this sequence to activate all the body's systems. The postures stimulate circulation, remove wastes and toxins and leave you feeling energised.

164

Practise this sequence when you are finding it difficult to stay **focused.** The postures will **balance** out the left and right sides of your body and help develop **concentration** and **willpower.**

Focus and balance

1. *Tadasana,* page 28

2. *Vrksasana,* page 30

3. *Virabhadrasana II,* page 38

4. *Ardha Chandrasana,* page 42

5. *Garudasana,* page 50

6. *Dandasana,* page 62

7. *Adho Mukha Svanasana,* page 100

8. *Urdhva Mukha Svanasana,* page 92

9. *Salamba Sarvangasana,* page 104

10. Forward Rest, page 122

11. *Virasana* Meditation page 134

12. *Savasana I,* page 110

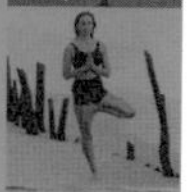

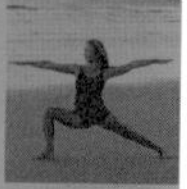

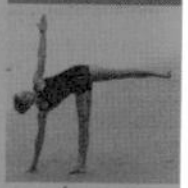

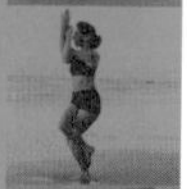

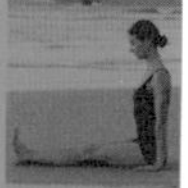

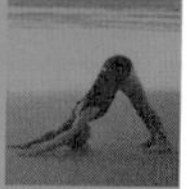

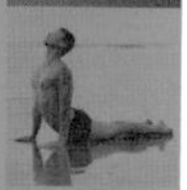

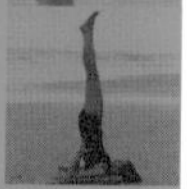

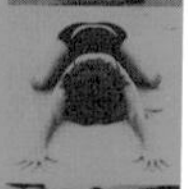

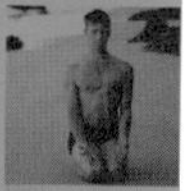

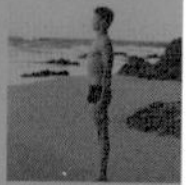

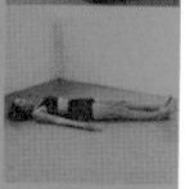

Relieving backache

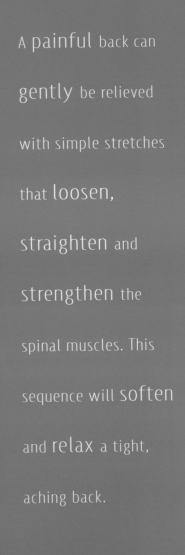

A painful back can gently be relieved with simple stretches that loosen, straighten and strengthen the spinal muscles. This sequence will soften and relax a tight, aching back.

A strong stomach helps to support the back and promotes good posture. This sequence also tones the internal organs, stimulating good digestion and bodily functions.

Abdominal toning

1. *Virasana I*, page 72

2. *Virasana II*, page 74

3. Greeting the day: three times, page 138

4. *Trikonasana*, page 32

5. *Janu Sirsasana*, page 68

6. *Navasana*: three times, page 78

7. *Salabhasana*, page 94

8. Mini Backbend, page 96

9. Knee Hug, page 120

10. *Salamba Sarvangasana*, page 104

11. Sitting with the breath, page 22

12. *Savasana II*, page 112

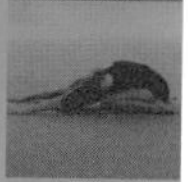

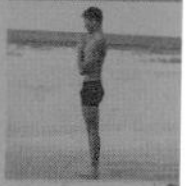

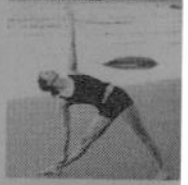

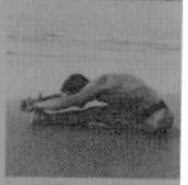

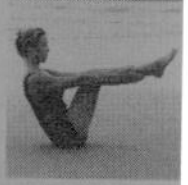

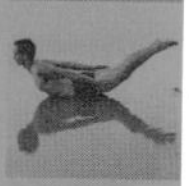

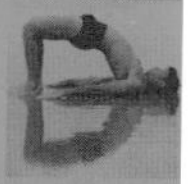

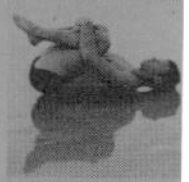

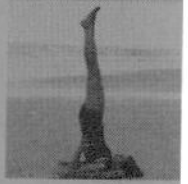

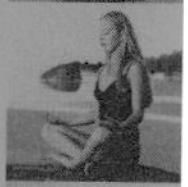

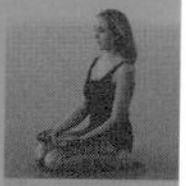

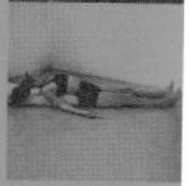

Toning the reproductive system

Healthy sexual organs, muscles and glands resist disease and help balance hormone levels in the body. Practise this sequence to keep the reproductive system functioning well.

These relaxing postures relieve agitation or stress experienced during menopause. The postures are designed to cool the body and calm the mind.

Relieving menopause

1. Inverted Legs I, page 102

2. Inverted Legs II, page 102

3. Inverted Legs III, page 102

4. Greeting the day: once, page 138

5. *Urdhva Mukha Svanasana*, page 92

6. *Janu Sirsasana*: with head on bolster, page 68

7. *Tri' Muk' Pas'*: with head on pillow, page 70

8. *Salamba Sarvangasana*, page 104

9. Forward Rest, page 122

10. Sitting with the breath, page 22

11. *Savasana I*, page 110

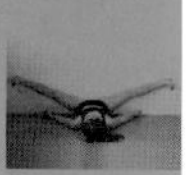

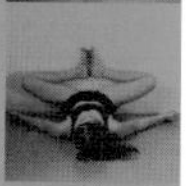

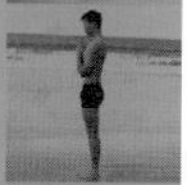

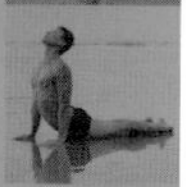

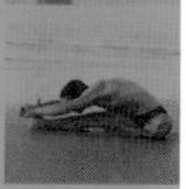

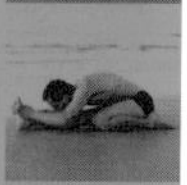

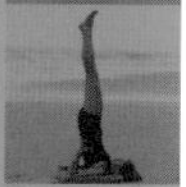

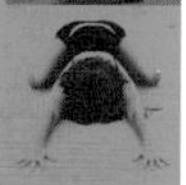

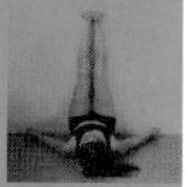

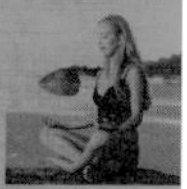

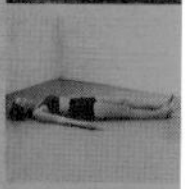

Evening wind-down

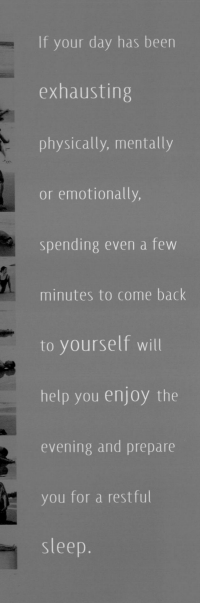

If your day has been

exhausting

physically, mentally

or emotionally,

spending even a few

minutes to come back

to yourself will

help you enjoy the

evening and prepare

you for a restful

sleep.

Headache can be caused by many factors, such as stress, fear, tiredness or menstruation. This sequence will gently stimulate circulation and relax the body and mind, helping to relieve an aching head.

Relieving headache

1. *Savasana II*, page 112

2. *Supta Baddha Konasana*, page 116

3. Forward Rest, page 122

4. *Janu Sirsasana*: with head resting on pillow, page 68

5. *Tri' Mukh' Pasc'*: with head resting on pillow, page 70

6. *Bharadvajrasana*, page 82

7. *Maricyasana* Twist, page 84

8. Child Pose, page 118

9. Inverted Legs I, page 102

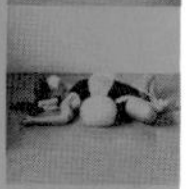

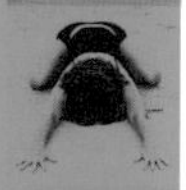

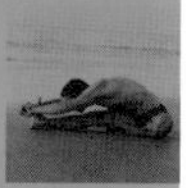

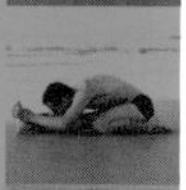

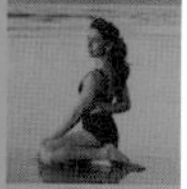

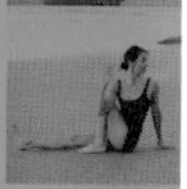

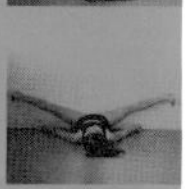
10. Inverted Legs II, page 102

11. Sitting with the breath, page 22

12. *Savasana II*: with eye bag, page 112

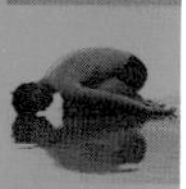

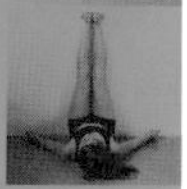

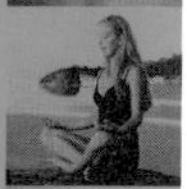

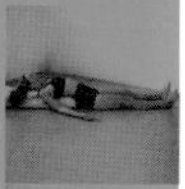

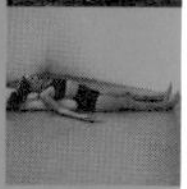

The following beginner's courses are made up of a sequence of postures from this book, combining standing, sitting, twisting, backbending, inverted and relaxation *asanas*. Some courses have a certain focus. For example, standing postures teach balance and twisting postures release toxins and soften the spine. All of the courses include standing and sitting postures and conclude with relaxation. Always finish with a version of *Savasana* or another relaxation posture for at least five minutes.

These sessions are your own private yoga classes and are a great way to explore the yoga postures. Each course is designed to be about thirty minutes long.

It is ideal to practise yoga every day for a healthy mind and body. However, three sessions a week is sufficient to keep your body toned and flexible throughout the week.

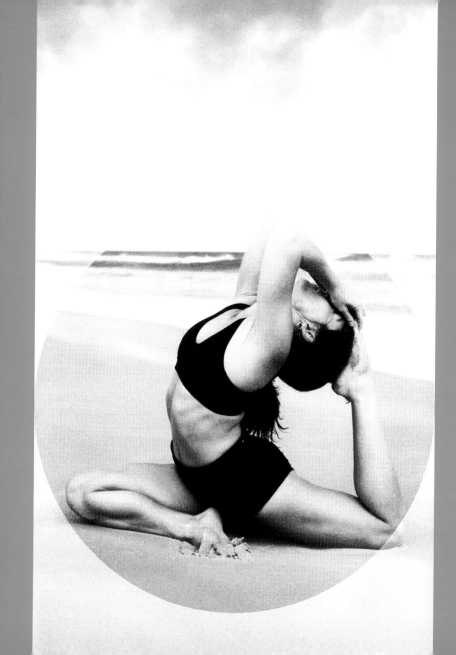

General yoga courses

Course One

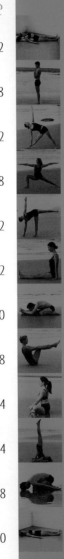

Course Two

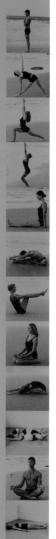

Course Three

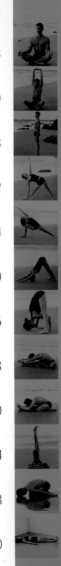

Course Four

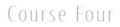
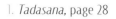
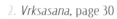
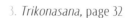
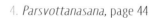
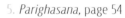
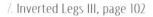

Course Five

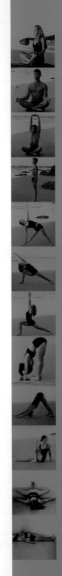

Course Six

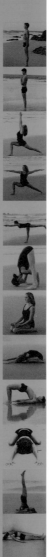

Course Seven

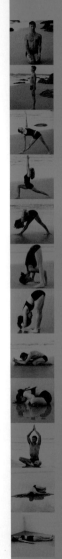

Course Eight

Course Nine

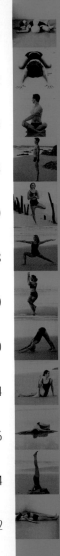

Course Ten

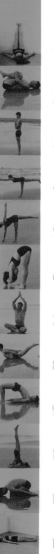

Course Eleven

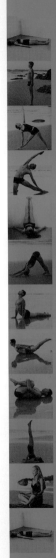

Course Twelve

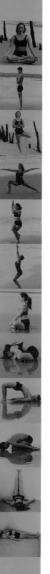

Course Thirteen

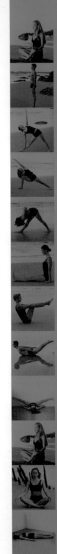

Course Fourteen

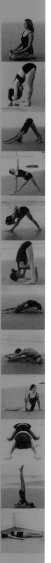

Course Fifteen

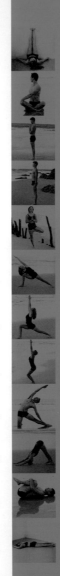

Course Sixteen

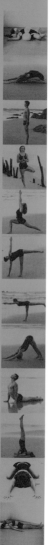

Course Seventeen

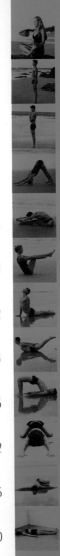

Course Eighteen

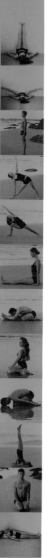

Index

About the author

Jessie grew up on the north coast of New South Wales in a bush house set in lush rainforest. At the age of twenty-two, after travelling for three years, she returned to Australia with a renewed interest in living a simple life and having a limited impact on the natural environment.

Jessie first started to practise yoga postures in 1991, exploring the effects yoga has on the body and mind, and observing how it brings out the best in people. She learnt under many dedicated teachers who enriched her passion for yoga and her understanding of it. Jessie went on to study and work in various healing arts, recognising in yoga the key to living a healthy and harmonious life. In 1997–98 she studied a yoga teacher training course with Louisa Sear from *Yoga Arts* in Byron Bay.

Yoga has been an enormous source of enjoyment in Jessie's life. This has inspired her to record her experiences to encourage beginners in the art of yoga.

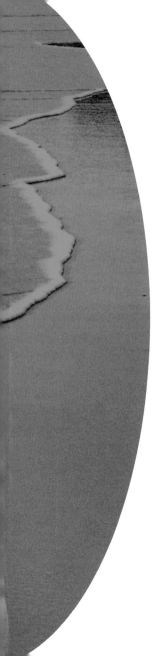

About the photographer

Dhyan divides his time between Byron Bay, Indonesia and the Philippines. He has an enormous passion for life, adventure, experience and people, and this love of exploration has led him to many different peoples, cultures and worlds. His talents include photography, surfing, building, travelling, music and art.

Photography is one of Dhyan's favourite creative outlets. His photographic collection includes whales and dolphins playing in the seas at Byron Bay, people from many cultures, and landscapes of breathtaking beauty. Dhyan's quest for spirituality is reflected in his collection of photos of monasteries in Tibet, ashrams in India, gurus from many different teachings and in his images of the Buddha.

Dhyan loves to photograph the body in yoga *asanas*. His photos aim to capture the essence of yoga.

Acknowledgments

Making this book has been an exciting journey, especially when working with yoga models. Their patience when modelling postures in wet sand and in freezing temperatures wearing very little was extraordinary. Thanks so much to you all: Rachel Hull (yogaroom@yahoo.com), Louisa Sear (yogarts@hotmail.com), Mathew James (yogamat@yahoo.com), Peter Watkins (Watkins@mullum.com.au), Ronit Robbaz Franco (Nitro117@hotmail.com) and Aloka.

Special thanks to Dhyan for all the time and energy he put into creating the beautiful photographs that capture the essence of the postures.

Thanks to my mother Carole and sister Judy for their inspiration and support.

Thanks also to all the yoga teachers I have learnt from, who have contributed their unique gifts and enhanced my experience of yoga over the years.

Finally, I wish to thank the people who made it possible. To the HarperCollins team: Helen Littleton, for sharing my vision; Jane Morrow and Wendy Blaxland, the editors who pulled it all together; and Katie Mitchell for her stunning design and layout of the book. Thanks also to Dr Arne Rubenstein for his contribution and to Mark Surman for his help with the photography.

Further reading

If you want to further your understanding of yoga postures, relaxation and meditation, try the following books:

T.K.V. Desikachar, *The Heart of Yoga: Developing a Personal Practice*, 1999, Inner Traditions Intl Ltd.

B.K.S. Iyengar, *The Art of Yoga*, (out of print – try your local library or a second-hand bookshop).

B.K.S. Iyengar and Yeudi Menuhin *Light on Yoga: Yoga Dipika*, 1995, Schocken Books.

Annie Jones, *Yoga: A Step-by-Step Guide*, 1998, Element.

Silva Mehta, Mira Mehta and Shyam Mehta, *Yoga: The Iyengar Way*, 1990, Knopf.

Mary Stewart and Maxine Tobias, *The Yoga Book*, 1986, Pan.

Selvarajan Yesudian, *Yoga Week by Week*, (out of print – try your local library or a second-hand bookshop).

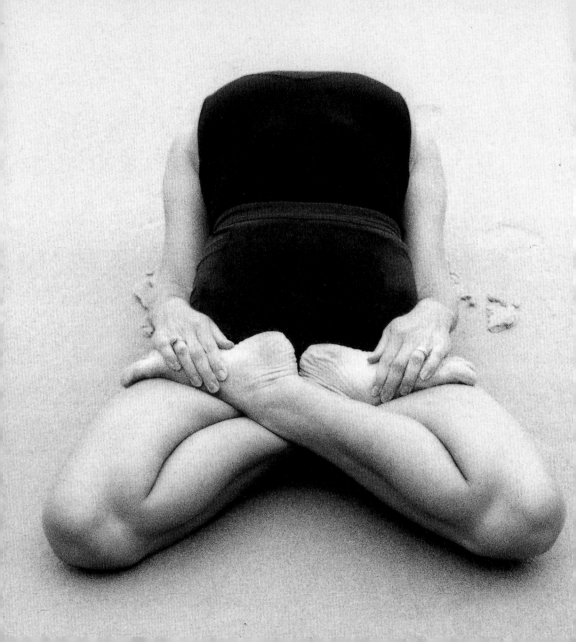